JOURNEY TO JUSTICE

DATE DUE

Library of Congress Catalog
Card Number 88-71206
ISBN 0-9620549-0-9

Back Cover Photo: Zane Williams

Additional copies of *Journey to Justice* may be ordered from:
Catalyst, P.O. Box 20572, Sarasota, Florida 34238-3572.

Printed in the United States of America
Printing: 1 2 3 4 5 6 7 8 9

Diane Craig Chechik

Editor
Eleanor S. Anderson

A Woman's True Story
of Breast Cancer
and Medical Malpractice

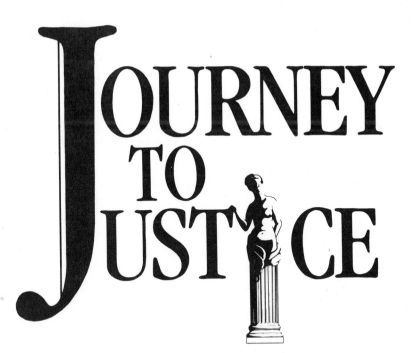

JOURNEY TO JUSTICE

catalyst

Sarasota, Florida

To Marc and Joel, my sons, whose support, courage, laughter, good judgment, love, and spirit for life and justice encouraged me not to falter. And to my dad, Maury (1908–1957), and mom, Dorothy Craig, for their faith in me.

ACKNOWLEDGMENTS

Thanks, first, to Eleanor Anderson, my editor and my loyal friend. Ellie has breast cancer. Dr. Paul Carbone is her oncologist, and we share the love and respect for the University of Wisconsin Clinical Cancer Center and its staff. I do not think anyone else could have edited this book. She kept my mission on target. Our close relationship and her experience with cancer and chemotherapy gave her unique insight and empathy for my story. Ellie often said, "Stick with me, you won't go wrong." Dear Ellie, thank you for the opportunity to stick with you. I plan to do just that for many years.

Thanks also to the many people who encouraged me (some relentlessly) to tell this story and who have supported me throughout:

My network, including Aviva Woll, Penny Aronson, and Judy Mostovoy, friends from school days in Chicago; Shirley Roskin, my college sorority roommate; and Mom and Dad Chechik, Uncle George and Aunt "Nish" Finer, Felice Levin, George Bush, Gail Chechik Wenocur, Herb and Frieda Cohn, Sidney Carpenter, Mom, Evan and Jane Pizer, Kay Gale, Sue Engstrom, J. darwin Yokum, Beth Rasmussen, Margo Ahrens, Bette McCaulley, Bonnie Paul, Pat McClure, and Sandy Larson.

All my lawyers, including Bill Smoler, who represented me in my malpractice case; Robert M. Callagy of New York City, whose expertise was invaluable in the preparation of this book; and in Madison, Dick Kabaker, who always raises my spirits with his comment that "anyone having me do their estate has automatic longevity"; Tim Valentyn, who taught me the value of patience as we began working to get this book published; and Howie Goldberg, who guided me through my personal court battles.

My sons, Marc and Joel, who edited the first draft and put my ideas into some kind of order; and Lynn and Ann Long, who spent long hours on the word processor to produce my first manuscript.

Linda Neu, who listened when no one else would, even when "it was real boring."

Readers of the revised manuscript, including Sandy Larson, Fred Coleman, Dick Kabaker, Bill Smoler, Robert M. Callagy, Rorie Craven Shefferman, Dr. Paul Carbone, and Helen Baldwin, who also helped me with several ventures for the University of Wisconsin Clinical Cancer Center. (A portion of the proceeds from the sale of each book will go to the University of Wisconsin Clinical Cancer Center through the University of Wisconsin Foundation's Bascom Hill Society.)

Mom, for living through this.

And, thank God for the telephone. It was a lifeline to friends.

Diane Craig Chechik
August 1987

CONTENTS

PREFACE

The impact of cancer on someone's life is not often revealed even to me, a physician who must advise patients about their illness and treatment. Patients come to me with fear, anger, and depression, having been told they have cancer by their general physician. Very often they come with families: mothers, daughters, sons, grandchildren, husbands, or wives. I go over the records, look at the pathology slides, and examine the patients. I spend 20 to 40 minutes in this process. Sometimes I ask to do additional tests, but more often than not I can come up with a plan. With just a minimum of interaction I must tell the patient that he or she has cancer, that it is serious or not serious, and that we do or do not have therapy to offer.

Inevitably I get asked, "How long do I have to live?" The answer I feel most comfortable giving is that percentages don't mean much for any one individual. A 20 percent chance of rain does not mean one could get 20 percent wet. One either gets wet or doesn't. The struggle against cancer in a single patient will result in 100 percent cure or 100 percent death. Therefore statistics are hard to apply to individuals. I do not understand how physicians can tell individual patients that they have six and one-half months or years to live. I am astounded daily by the many patients who beat the odds, or by people who should have everything in their favor yet fail and develop metastatic cancer early. We still have many things to learn about this disease and more to learn about the inner strength of people who face its threats. I usually tell them that cancer, unlike heart disease, does not strike people down quickly and that the end will not be a surprise. It is important to tell people that you as a physician will be there to help them. Initially you will give them specific treatments for their cancer, but later you will be there helping them to stave off pain or vomiting or fear. They must have a sense that you will be with them. They must not be abandoned because you have run out of drugs, X-ray treatments, or surgeries. I tell my students that if one enters medicine primarily to cure people, one goes into obstetrics. That is one of the few "illnesses" that can be cured. Most of the rest of medical practice involves helping people live successfully with their problems or treating the symptoms. We can and do cure cancer but as cancer specialists we must be prepared to treat and care for our patients totally as humans worthy of our ministrations.

In this book Diane Craig Chechik pours out her emotions fully, detailing her struggles as a unique individual to preserve her self-image. She trusts people but has a need to be convinced in a logical manner. She is able to survive by maintaining an independent mind and philosophy. She has a strong sense of justice. Her struggles in the doctors' offices, the treatment rooms, and the law courts are all laid out in strong personal tones. She knows how to get the answers. She is persistent. This kind of person has a very positive effect on others who need direction and advice in how to handle their struggles. Diane's descriptions of the chemotherapy, the side effects, and the fears of therapy are all laid out. I suspect that if she had a serious heart problem or kidney disease she would do the same thing. While she describes her family support systems, it is clear that she was struggling not only against her cancer but in her personal life for some quality and reason. She fought this fight on her own. It would be important and interesting to learn the impact of cancer on the lives of the spouses, children, friends, and lovers of cancer patients.

The messages that come from this book are many. First, knowledge about the body and its illnesses is an important aid one has in seeking the right opinions. Cancer occurs in many shapes and forms. Most lumps are not cancer, but lumps must be observed carefully or diagnosed accurately. Regular self-examination of the breasts can detect early problems. Mammograms are helpful in the diagnosis of cancer, but even that test is not always right. Treatment needs to be aggressive and participation in clinical trials may often be the right therapy. While the generalist can do most things, second opinions are important and necessary.

Second, the struggle against cancer must involve the family of the patient, even though the patient is very often able to cope successfully with this serious illness. Finally, the patient must feel that she or he has some control in the matter. The pysche is stronger than one thinks. Explanations must be complete and yet simple. One must allow the patient time to think and talk issues over with others. There must be participation by the patient in the battle against cancer.

While every patient with cancer is not going to cope by writing a book, Diane had to do this. It is the way she copes. I admire her energy and the forthright way she has confronted life's problems and shared them with her readers.

Paul P. Carbone, M.D., F.A.C.P., D.Sc. (Hon.)
Director, University of Wisconsin Clinical Cancer Center
Professor and Chairman, Department of Human Oncology

PROLOGUE

"Diane Chechik went to Dr. Jackson for treatment. She trusted him. She believed in him. She's coming to you for justice."

With those words my attorney closed my case in a medical malpractice suit against Dr. C. R. Jackson of Madison, Wisconsin. It was November 1985. I felt I was finally at the end of a long ordeal, one that began more than three and one-half years before. From March 1982 until December 1983, Bob Jackson assured me three times that the lump in my breast was not cancer. In fact I was heading for a life-threatening crisis. Dr. Hiram Cody III of New York diagnosed my cancer on December 12, 1983—a date etched in my memory forever. It was the day my life changed. It was the day I began saying, "I have cancer." And it was the beginning of a painful course of treatment: a mastectomy, nearly a year of chemotherapy, removal of a new malignancy, and 30 treatments with radiation. Much of this might have been unnecessary if a proper diagnosis had been made in March 1982.

But it wasn't, and that fact made the lawsuit necessary. The odds were against me—I had only a two percent chance of winning the lawsuit. But that didn't stop me. I sued Bob Jackson for my sanity. He didn't do right. Justice had to be done.

This book is a journal of my ordeal—and of my journey into the worlds of breast cancer and justice. During much of that period I did not look or think like myself. I was confused. I couldn't concentrate. A few minutes spent on any one thing was too long. These were side effects of the medical procedures used to keep me alive. These procedures sometimes made me think and behave in strange ways. But my journal is published just as I wrote it. I do not apologize for the way I was then. I want readers to know what cancer patients and their loved ones go through.

I want this book to give others hope. Though there are easier ways for a person to grow, cancer is not a reason to give in to despair. My love of life holds me together. My love for my two boys, my mother, and my friends sees me through my new cancer world.

I keep this disease at bay with the help of medicine and especially with the extraordinary energy released in what I call my "cancer rage." I believe my cancer rage is a chemically produced state resulting from the medicines of chemotherapy. It strikes unexpectedly, causes extreme irritation, and shows itself in bursts of anger. My loved ones usually bear the brunt of my cancer rage. But those who know about it accept it, and the rage releases so much frustration that I have come to regard it as a friend.

I also fight despair by sitting under my Purple Tree. Yes, my Purple Tree. Everyone has a quiet place in the mind where they go when they are troubled. Frequently, during my ordeal, I would go and sit under my Purple Tree to gain the strength I needed to continue. My Purple Tree lets me dream and helps me achieve my dreams.

It would have been easy to allow this disease to wash over me, to leave me lethargic and inactive. But I'm not built that way. I've gone through life knowing I was someone different. I take risks; I'm a survivor. Survivors are a different breed.

All these things helped strengthen my determination to go through chemotherapy and radiation with class, with my sexuality intact, and most of all with a sense of humor. Life without those would be out of character for me. I had to do it this way. And I did.

There is a lot of help available to cancer patients. Nevertheless, the first lesson to learn is: Fight for yourself. It may be hard, but with your life at stake, you must start being selfish. Staying alive now, with my cancer treatment, is a full-time job. My family and friends felt threatened, at first, because of my new attitude that everything revolved around my disease. But my key to survival is to fight cancer every second, not to let it get to me for even a moment.

I know too that for me it is necessary to affirm that my head is connected to the rest of my body. Psychiatrists and psychologists can help provide some of the medicine you need. Unfortunately many people—doctors and insurance companies included—consider the head separately from the rest of the anatomy. But the right attitude is a positive and essential force in surviving this disease. I know my therapy has played an important part in my survival. I still have a good mind, and it still works.

The most important thing to learn from this book is courage. If you have or ever develop cancer, I hope you can find the courage to live proudly in your new world of cancer as a person with rights. You cannot sit on your hands and feel sorry for yourself. You cannot waste precious moments with that kind of negative thinking. Make yourself as beautiful as you can. Recognize you are fighting this battle alone, but that you can still call in your support troops when you need them.

Time is important to you. Make it your ally; don't fight it. Every new day that dawns for you means you're winning your fight for life. Your cancer and treatment will change you. Don't be afraid of it. You will not be the same as you were before cancer. In some ways you will be better.

This book begins with cancer and ends with my pursuit of justice. I still have cancer. My fight goes on. I continue to stretch myself physically and mentally beyond every conceivable limit to survive. My story is not over yet.

CHAPTER 1

March 29, 1982

I went to see Bob Jackson today. I had just found a lump on the outer side of my right breast. I was frightened. I thought I had cancer. Bob has been my doctor and friend for 16 years. I trust him. I was alone with him in the examining room. He said, "You certainly have a lump. We'll find out if it's a cyst. I don't think it's cancer." He took a needle aspiration of the lump. He held his hand carefully so he would be putting the needle into the middle of the lump. He pulled the needle out, laid it down on the counter, and said, "You're right. It's not a cyst. It's a lump." He told me to have a mammogram and not to worry about it; he didn't think it was cancer. I had a mammogram a few hours later.

Bob called this afternoon with the results of the mammogram. He said that everything is fine. He told me to continue my monthly breast examination and if anything changes to call him. He suggested I come back in three months. I asked him about a biopsy. He said, "No biopsy." That's what I wanted to hear. I was relieved. I trust him. He is my doctor and my friend.

June 29, 1982

I went back to Bob today. I told him nothing had changed. The lump is still there. I asked him what we should do about it. I told him I'm planning to leave tomorrow for a vacation in Salt Lake City, Utah, and I want to make sure I don't have cancer. I had another mammogram. He called this afternoon and told me everything was fine. "See, I told you not to worry. You are fine. You can live with it. It is not cancer." I again mentioned a biopsy. He said it was absolutely not necessary. He told me to forget everything—my lump and my divorce—and have a good time. Again he reminded me to continue the monthly breast examination and if anything did change to come right in. Otherwise, he said, he would see me at the usual time—between a year and 18 months.

Maybe I'm too conscious of cancer. Everyone on my father's side, including my father, died of cancer, although my father was not diagnosed as having it. Bob knows the fear I have of dying of cancer. He knows I'm afraid of having breast cancer before I'm 50 years old. But I trust him. He's been my good friend as well as my doctor. He's always been straight with me. We've had a successful doctor/patient relationship.

July 2, 1982

I came to Salt Lake City with Irving, as planned. I'm visiting a dear friend, Sidney Carpenter, and seeing my beloved mountains of Snowbird, Utah. I had Sidney feel the lump. Bob was her doctor when she lived in Madison. Irving also felt it, more than just in Utah. He is a feeling, active lover.

Then I decided to forget about it and enjoy my vacation. There's still a needle mark on my breast from the aspiration. I've decided not to pay attention, not to think about cancer. However, I *will* feel the lump every day to see if it changes.

March 9, 1983

Today I went to a doctor for the first time since last June. I went because I've just started working for a large insurance company and a physical exam is required.

This particular doctor, Blake Waterhouse, is a friend of Bob's and, I believe, a good doctor. I chose him because he is also a friend of mine; our children go to school together. Besides, he was the only doctor I knew on the list provided by the company. He examined me and asked what I was doing about the lump in my breast. I told him what Bob had said and done. He just raised his hand as if waving the whole thing away and said, "I defer to him." Then he went on to something else. Even though I was not there for diagnostic purposes, I did accept this as another opinion, along with the mammograms and Bob's assurances that my lump was not cancer.

November 1, 1983

Today I found a lump under my arm. Damn. Now I have two lumps. I think I have cancer. I walked into the living room after my bath and told my kids that I have breast cancer. "This time," I said, "it has spread." The boys said, "Here we go again. Oh Mom, you don't have cancer." I told myself, "This time I'm right. Son of a bitch."

Then I calmed down. Maybe the boys are right. I must have pulled a muscle playing tennis. And, it could be that it's just before my period and everything is different.

November 11, 1983

My mother, Dorothy Craig, went into the hospital today. She has some sort of infection around her heart. I cannot deal with this and the possibility of cancer at the same time. I haven't called my doctor yet. I figure a few more days won't make any difference anyway. Mom is my concern right now.

November 15, 1983

Mom almost died today. But she survived—as I prayed she would. This is not the first time she has gone through this scenario. I know she has a fantastic will to live. She's been through heart surgery twice already. The first surgery, a valve repair by Dr. William Young, was in 1966 at University of Wisconsin Hospital. In 1981 Mom went into University Hospital again, that time for a valve replacement by Dr. David Meyerowitz. He saved her life. While in the hospital she suffered cardiac arrest, kidney failure, and lung collapse. She almost suffered tracheotomy strangulation as well. All that 10 days after my divorce. And now this. I wonder: are Mom's medical crises timed by someone higher up to test me just when I'm experiencing a crisis?

When Mom was in the hospital in 1981, she experienced death and came back. One of my aunts and I took notes of her conversation as she slipped into another world. We listened to this remarkable woman tell us where she was going on her white horse. She told everyone goodbye. She told me she was sorry about causing me so much heartache. She said she had a mission to do all by herself and could not take me or anyone else with her. She had to go alone but told me not to worry because she would be seeing people she hadn't seen in a long time. She said she loved everyone in the family. I was to take care of the boys. She loved her grandchildren. Some day she would see them again. Then she said goodbye and went into a coma.

Her kidneys had shut down. The doctor and I decided not to put her on dialysis because it would be too hard and painful. She would die either way. Let her go in peace. She did not want life support; she had made me promise not to have them do any more. I signed the autopsy consent. I said goodbye to her. The doctors encouraged me to leave. There was nothing more to do. They would call me. Her sisters were there. I went home to wait for the call. The family talked about having a memorial service at my house. Mom did not want one in a church or temple even though she had a very strong belief in God.

At about three in the afternoon the hospital called and asked us to come down. Mom's kidneys had started again. She was awake. She was put on a lung machine. Mom was going to make it—we hoped.

This time I'm different with Mom's illness. I have to take care of myself. I have done all I can as a daughter.

November 21, 1983

It's my mother's birthday—one we hadn't been sure she'd be here to celebrate. We had a happy party, complete with a cake and flowers, in her hospital room.

Afterwards, it was time for me to take care of myself. I went to see Bob again. I told him I wanted a biopsy with Dr. John Pellett at University Hospital. I told him again that I believe I have cancer. He said, "You don't have cancer. You're jumping the gun and I'm not going to have you have a biopsy. You don't need it. It's a little pulled muscle. Don't worry. We'll watch it for 10 days after your period and then we'll see about it. It will probably go away the same way it came."

"No," I said, "I think it's cancer."

He said, "Relax. You don't have cancer."

November 29, 1983

Mother is getting better, and Felice, my good friend in New York, has invited me to visit. I began making plans today. I'll leave for New York on December 6.

December 8, 1983

I've been here in New York since Tuesday. I've been to several parties, including one given today by Felice and her husband, Harry. After the party, I told Felice about the lump in my breast. She's convinced me that I ought to see her breast doctor. He's considered one of the finest in the country. With much reservation I said, "Well, why not get another opinion?" I feel it won't hurt Bob's reputation if everything turns out okay. If it doesn't, that's a problem I'd rather not think about.

December 12, 1983

At 1 o'clock this afternoon I saw Dr. Hiram Cody III. He performed a needle biopsy. He nicked a blood vessel, which started to bleed, and this famous New York doctor couldn't find the right bandage. We both laughed. It was much-needed comic relief. He sent me to have a mammogram and an ultrasonic test.

Later in the afternoon I went back to his office. It was raining hard. He said very simply, "Diane, you have breast cancer and lymph node involvement. You are in Stage Two.

"In Stage Two, your chances for survival, your treatment, and your chances for recurrence are all different. In March and June 1982, you were most likely at Stage One."

The words rang in my head. I could hear thunder from the storm outside. It was *nothing* compared to the storm building inside me.

He continued, "Your life is in danger; you're too young." I heard him speak, but I didn't know what all his words meant.

He told me I could have a mastectomy here in New York or at the University of Wisconsin Hospital in Madison. "But," he repeated, "you must have it immediately. Time is essential." He told me I would be in chemotherapy and maybe radiation. He told me how the mastectomy had to be done for the cancer not to spread more. I listened. I grasped at every word of encouragement he had for me. There were very few. I listened with fear. I was going to die. I wanted people I loved around me. There was no one.

I have breast cancer. My greatest fear is now reality. My mind raced through the events of the last 20 months. Why did

Bob keep assuring me, "Diane, you don't have cancer"? Why would he not do a biopsy when I kept asking him to do one? It wasn't easy to tell Dr. Cody that my doctor in Madison had never done a biopsy. Twenty months were crucial.

I guess I really did hear what Dr. Cody was saying, though, because I finally told him, "They're not going to get me." He told me I didn't have a choice about the surgery. We were talking about my life.

At that moment I knew Dr. Hiram Cody III saved my life.

I left Dr. Cody's office and met Felice. When I told her his diagnosis, we hugged and cried. Then we left the building and went to have a drink. Scotch was all I could swallow. I was cold sober, but I was dazed. It was like a nightmare.

We came back here to Felice's apartment. The storm had gotten worse outside as well as inside my head and my heart. It was 4 o'clock in the afternoon when I called Bob Jackson. I wanted him to make plans for me to go to the hospital. I had decided, and Dr. Cody agreed, that being in Madison, my home, would be better than being in New York for the surgery. I need everyone around me: my boys, my family, and my friends.

When I got Bob's office on the phone, his nurse told me he was with a patient. I told her I didn't care: this was an emergency. He came to the phone and said, "Well, what is it, Diane, that is so important?"

"Bob, I have breast cancer. I am in Stage Two and my life is in danger. I have to have surgery Friday and I want Dr. John Pellett to do it."

"You don't have cancer," he said. "What the hell are you doing in New York seeing another doctor?"

I told him that I had gone to see one of the finest breast doctors in the country for another opinion.

He said, "I'll bet you $100 you don't have cancer and that it will go away. You get back here, get your stuff and your records, and I will tell you that you don't have cancer. Just get home. I will see you on Wednesday. You do not have cancer."

"Goodbye, Bob," I said, and hung up.

I could not believe this was happening to me. Why would Bob still not believe I have cancer? Why did he insist that he is right and my "New York doctor" and I are wrong? It's pouring rain outside, but there are more tears in my eyes. Right now I don't know how I can continue another day, another hour, another minute, knowing I have cancer.

Strange as it seems, I was hungry. I could still eat. All was not lost! And all I wanted was barbecued spareribs. So Felice, Harry, and I walked to a nearby restaurant for dinner and I had my ribs.

I can think of little else but Dr. Cody's diagnosis of cancer and the phone call to Bob Jackson. Son of a bitch! I feel betrayed.

My thoughts aren't coherent. I'm fighting for my life. I must tell my boys. I'm alone. I have cancer. I'm dying. I'm too young to die. I'll fight like hell to live.

I've finished off a little more Scotch tonight, but I'm still sober. How will I get through the next 24 hours? What else? I'll go Christmas shopping. This might be my last time and my last Christmas. Christ, I can't let myself think like that. That cancer bastard is not going to get me down!

December 13, 1983

As I expected, I didn't get much sleep last night. Even the Scotch didn't help. I thought about many things—good and bad—during those long, sleepless hours. I love New York. I remembered that New York was where I had come up with the idea of creating Catalyst, Inc., my interior design boutique. New York was where I had tried to save my marriage. And now it might be the place that saves my life. I thought of one of the lines from the song "New York, New York"—"If I make it here, I'll make it anywhere."

I *am* going to make it, here in New York City and everywhere. I *am* going to live. *I will survive.*

As if to taunt me, the first thing I saw on the breakfast table this morning was a *New York Times* headline that read: "Divorce Stress Exacts Long-Term Health Toll." Among other things, reporter Jane Brody pointed out that ". . .compared with married, never-married and widowed, divorced adults have higher rates of emotional disturbances, accidental death and death from heart disease, cancer. . . ." It's as if she wrote it just for me.

I did go shopping today. Then I picked up my medical records and had lunch at the Overseas Press Club. Felice insisted that I have a steak sandwich. She called it "my last good meal before all hell breaks loose." Not quite the Last Supper. And then I took off for Madison. I wonder if I'll ever see Felice again. But I shouldn't think like that. I'll face the unknown with strength.

My son Marc met me at the airport. He told me he was submitting a proposal to change jobs at his company. He thought it was quite good. He said if it wasn't accepted he would quit. He graduated last year from the University of Missouri with a degree in journalism. He wants to write, produce, and do something more than sell advertising for a magazine. He read his proposal to me at dinner. I told him my opinion and that he had done a good job.

Then I took a deep breath and, taking his hand, I told him about the events of the last 24 hours. I told him I have cancer. I told him not to tell his brother until tomorrow after his final exam.

December 14, 1983

I drove through a snowstorm to Bob's office. At first he was very curt. Then he examined me and said, "I guess you do have cancer." He called Dr. Cody in New York and was very sweet to him. Bob thanked him for taking such good care of me. I tried to relate his cordiality and charm to his angry words to me just 48 hours earlier. He got the results of all my tests. Everything that Dr. Cody said about the breast cancer was now verified.

He came around his desk to me and started to cry. He said, "Oh, my God, what have I done to you?" He closed the office door, and we both cried. He then told me we would get through this together. His words made little sense, but we were both so emotional that I was confused about what I heard.

He said he'd make all the arrangements with Dr. John Pellett at University Hospital for my admission tomorrow. I requested Dr. Pellett because I had heard he was excellent. Bob told me to go home and stay there. He would call me with the information. He also told me he was awfully glad I was going to have my surgery before he goes on vacation to Hawaii. I left his office and started driving to my mother's apartment. I wanted her arms around me. I was scared. I was angry. I felt betrayed again. I felt lost. This is going to be one fight I *have* to win.

I drove with tears in my eyes. I'll be in the hospital tomorrow.

Mom greeted me with her wonderful smile. She said, "You're here. That's great." I went in, closed the door, put my head on her chest, and cried. I told her I have cancer. She held me in her arms and we both cried. I told her about the mastectomy Friday. I told her that my life is in danger. This is the great woman who has had two open heart surgeries. She's a miracle. She's been my guiding light.

"Diane," she said, "we are from tough stuff. You'll make it too." She put her arms around me again and said, "Nah, you're not going to die. We've got a lot of living to do."

When I got home I called several people. Then I burst into tears again, this time in Marc's arms. Now I had to call Joel. He had just finished one final exam and had one more to go. I told him I thought he had better come home. He was studying and said, "Well, I really don't think I can."

I said, "I think you'd best come home now."

"Aw, come on, Mom."

I took a deep breath and said, "Joel, I have cancer and I'm going in for a mastectomy tomorrow. I must see you tonight."

I don't know how he got there, but it seemed like just five minutes later he was at the door. I opened the door and burst into tears. Joel and I just held one another. Marc walked over and the three of us just cried. "You'll make it, Mom. We'll be with you," they said. We talked. We cried. I need my boys.

I called my friend Kay. I called Al, my former husband. They both came over. Then Bob called and gave me the details about checking into the hospital.

December 15, 1983

Before I left for the hospital today I made cookies. Making chocolate chip cookies on the first and last day of school each semester is a family tradition begun when Marc started kindergarten in 1964. Today was the last day of finals at the UW-Madison, where Joel is a sophomore.

So I carried on, even though I was about to have major surgery and my life was in danger. There were tears in my eyes. Maybe in the cookies too.

Then I came to the hospital. When I was settled in my room, my "precious friend" Dr. George Bush came to see me. He said he would take care of me. George is a cancer patient too. He held my hand and told me what to expect from surgery.

I've known George since 1974, when he and his first wife were my clients at Catalyst, Inc. Of course, I knew he was a doctor. I thought he was a gastroenterologist. Imagine my surprise, then, when he announced that he would be my anesthetist tomorrow. "What?! But you're a gastroenterologist. Since when do you give anesthetics?"

"Since before I met you at Catalyst," George said. "It's been my specialty all along." He explained that the anesthetist I had requested couldn't change her schedule, so he'd be substituting.

Dr. Pellett was here too. He told me what he'll be doing tomorrow. He was gentle, precise, and calming. I haven't really had time to think about what it will mean to have only one breast. I did ask two friends who've had mastectomies about that. One is Aviva Meyers Woll, a friend from Sullivan High School days in Chicago. She had the surgery about a year ago. The other friend, who lives in Madison, had surgery a couple of years ago. Both said it wasn't so bad. And Aviva said she'd be up to see me on Sunday.

It's been too cold for Mom to come to the hospital. But I've talked to her on the phone several times today. We need each other. We're both saying a lot of prayers.

And that reminds me of an amusing incident. I've always believed in God; praying is not new to me. And now I know I'll have to depend on my faith more than ever. When I checked into the hospital, they asked me about my religion. I said, "All." I was told that wouldn't go into the computer. So they read all the religions listed in their computer. When they came to "Other," I said, "That's it, Other."

Bob came to see me. He said he was sorry, that he had made a terrible mistake. He said he doesn't know why he didn't do a biopsy. He said he had goofed. He said that he should never have relied only on a mammogram. He said he should have done more.

I stared in disbelief. Again, his words made little sense. I did not contradict anything he said. I could not. My trust in Bob is gone.

CHAPTER 2

December 17, 1983

I came through the operation okay yesterday. I'm still alive. There are no complications from the mastectomy. It was not just a bad dream. It was real. I was terrified. I haven't had time yet to think about what all this will mean in my life.

When I opened my eyes after surgery, I saw George looking down at me. He was also the last person I saw before surgery. He had told me a joke as he administered the anesthetic. I was smiling as I went to sleep. When I woke up he said everything was okay. His smiling eyes and the security in his voice gave me a minute of peace. He held my hand and told me he would visit me later and tell me the joke again.

When I awoke a second time I was in my room. My dearest friend Kay was standing beside my bed and holding my hand. She said it was too cold outside for me to do anything anyway, so I might as well stay where I was and get well. She talked about our ski trip to Snowbird, Utah, in eight weeks. She knew more than her smile revealed. After all, Kay is a fine doctor.

Soon the boys were here. They had been told I would not be down for a long time, so they had gone to lunch. I surprised them. I came back early. I held their hands and I slept.

December 20, 1983

It's been four days since the surgery. Today it was time to take the bandages off and see what all this means.

Since the operation a special nurse has spent a lot of time with me. She is Sandy Larson, head supervisor nurse for chemotherapy. She came to meet me and to talk about some aspects of the treatment I'll be receiving. I liked her instantly. She's smiling, smart, and sincere—my kind of woman. What a special lady!

I asked her to be with me when John Pellett took the bandages off. I needed her to hold my hand. I needed her reassurance. I thought I was ready to deal with what was under the bandages. But a little extra support couldn't hurt. Dr. John Pellett and Sandy Larson—two special people helping me start my new life.

Reality is the day the bandages come off. And when they came off, there was my new body. I didn't know how I would react. And my first words surprised even me. "That's beautiful," I said. "It's my life." I closed my eyes. I wanted to cry out, "It's not horrible. It's not ugly. It's just different." I held Sandy's hand so tightly that her fingers almost turned blue. I was scared.

"It looks terrific," Dr. Pellett said, and smiled. He feels it's truly a work of art. He's a sensitive man and takes great pride in his work. He left a little skin for my cleavage, and to help if I decide to have reconstruction. This, I decided, is a small price to pay for life.

It was the right decision to have Sandy here with me. I would suggest to every woman who has a mastectomy not to be alone when the bandages are taken off.

After Sandy and the doctor left, I looked down again. It *is* beautiful. It's certainly different, but it's still me. Everyone who goes through this operation must find her own way. I'm struggling to live. But accepting the situation as it exists—which I have begun to do—is going to make that battle a lot easier to win.

When Marc first saw the scar, he said he thought it was beautiful. "A fine work of art," he called it. "John's a fine surgeon." Joel agreed but didn't say too much. He was more concerned about the health of his mother than about the loss of her breast. Their sensitivity is heart-warming. They have grown up.

December 21, 1983

Al came to see me. I could feel his coldness and, strangely, his annoyance at the situation.

My boys are terrified at the events of the last 10 days. Even my mother, courageous lady that she is, isn't sure what to do next. This strong woman saw for the first time that her daughter was sicker than she was. She did all she could. She's been a wonderful mother. I have taken care of her in her various illnesses. Now the roles are reversed. As sick as I am, I have the feeling that people are depending on me to give them strength, courage, and direction.

December 23, 1983

I'm leaving the hospital today, in time to celebrate Christmas at home. My heart's desire is for everything to be as it was just two short weeks ago. But in my head I know that I must accept what is. I *will*. Yesterday I was finally able to talk fairly calmly about the new me, but I don't know what to expect. I asked my new friend Sandy Larson to let me tape her impressions of me—how she felt about me and my reactions to the events of the last week. This is how she put it:

"I would like to backtrack a little. I would like to talk about the Diane that I first met in her hospital room. A Diane who needed to relax underneath an exterior of absolute sheer energy; who was spinning in every direction and no direction. She needed to stop the phone calls, stop the many visitors, and bring everything to a grinding halt.

"It was time to focus on the healing Diane—the inner Diane. Your energy was going in every direction, but not toward you. We talked about the center, which is really the core, and the outer circles around that core. We talked about having to focus into your own inner circle. I think that was really hard for you. You were frightened.

"We spent a great deal of time on that. How it was okay to be scared. And that sometimes a person just needs to let the tears out and cry, cry, cry.

"You were exhausted. You were struggling to reach the surface so you could grab the strength to keep yourself afloat. Your survival skills have more to do with your keeping right up on top and struggling to keep up that cheerful front—keeping your sense of humor, which is so important. For you it is one of the most important ingredients of being well and staying well.

"You have to be careful trying to stay 'up' too much. Sometimes when you are alone with me or someone else you can trust, you can let down. It's okay. It's necessary for healing.

"The day I held your hand, there was a different Diane. I saw you grow. After my second visit with you, when you were still struggling and grasping for that center inside the circle to hold onto, I think we developed a rapport with one another.

"It meant a great deal to me that you were able to ask me to be here with you when you had the bandages taken off. You were asking for help. I saw it as a beginning, because you couldn't do it all by yourself—not forever. You are a remarkable woman with remarkable drive and energy. You have a circle of friends who all feel for you. I knew it was a positive sign when you felt you needed some extra support. You needed it from a sensitive nurse—someone besides your doctor. The moment the bandages came off you were frightened and you clung to my hand—like a child afraid to look.

"I wish I had had a movie camera at that moment. Words just don't describe it. You looked down at yourself and your eyes would go only so far, then stop. Then you would look down again and your eyes would go only so far. Then they would go a little farther. It sounds like a long time; it was only a few minutes. It seemed like forever. Finally, you saw everything.

"That is where Diane changed. A peaceful Diane emerged. 'That's beautiful! That's me!' You began to take your hand to delicately caress the scar, the place where you used to have a breast. It was one of the most beautiful scenes of my life. It was the humanity of the situation. How beautiful you were—inside and out. A beautiful healing was taking place. It was becoming part of you and you welcomed it."

December 24, 1983

It's Christmas Eve. I've been home from the hospital since yesterday. Al will be here tonight. I thought it would be nice for the boys to have their father here. Who knows? It might be the last Christmas they have with me.

December 25, 1983

The four of us had a wonderful evening last night. At first. Al and I were getting along fine. We had a beautiful time sitting before the fire and playing games and music. The phone rang about 11:30. I answered it. It was the last of the many women Al had a relationship with during our married life. She is also his current lover. She wanted to talk with him. I went into hysterics. She had no right to call my house—ever—even though Al and I are divorced. It seemed like she couldn't stand the idea that he was with his family, even though I had just been home from the hospital for 24 hours.

Al talked with her briefly. Our boys were furious. He left, at his sons' request. I cried. Suddenly I knew I had to protect myself. Nothing must keep me from getting and staying well. I'm going to fight to stay alive.

All in all, it was not the happiest Christmas I have known.

CHAPTER 3

January 1, 1984

It's the beginning of a new year. The past three weeks have been the most unexpected—and scariest—of my life. I have a fairly active and fertile imagination. But 365 days ago even *I* could not have dreamed up what has happened to me since December 12—that I would be recuperating from a mastectomy and getting ready to begin a yearlong course of chemotherapy. My first treatment is January 5.

January 4, 1984

Tomorrow is the day I begin chemotherapy. I'm terrified. What will chemotherapy do to me? Even the doctors can't say for sure, because no two patients react exactly the same way. They hope it kills the cancer cells. It also kills good cells—generally the fastest-growing cells—which is why one of the most common side effects is the loss of hair.

Sandy Larson and my oncologists have tried their best to prepare me for what is to come. I'll be on a *protocol*—medical jargon for the combination of substances to be used in the course of treatment—that includes nine drugs. I'll be part of a study comparing the effects of these drugs to another group of drugs on premenopausal women with breast cancer. For one year I'll be on the highest doses of this protocol.

My surgeon, Dr. Pellett, pushed for this tougher protocol. He doesn't think the regular protocol will do the job. Although he feels he got it all, there is still the small, outside chance he missed something. He wants me to have every chance.

Dr. Paul Carbone, director of the University of Wisconsin Clinical Cancer Center, is involved in this study of 440 women. I've been told this protocol is tougher than most. But I fit the criteria for the study. So I gave my consent to be part of this test. I'm going into this with my eyes wide open.

January 5, 1984

The dreadful day has arrived. I'm terrified of chemotherapy. I'm terrified of having cancer. I'm terrified of living in my new world. And I'm terrified of dying. But I've psyched myself up to live, no matter what it takes. After all, the idea is to drive the malignancy out of my body and to keep me alive. I will not let this cancer bastard get me down.

I wore my white satin boa today when I went in for my first chemo treatment. It's a little gift I bought for myself after the mastectomy from Neiman-Marcus in Chicago. I charged it without even knowing the price. But that didn't matter since it was good for my health to have beauty and luxury around my new body. It's sexy. I feel beautiful wearing it.

Then I decided to wear it during my examinations at the hospital. The gowns they give you are asexual, to say the least. Just because I have one breast doesn't mean I need to look asexual and ugly.

I wore my boa today when I went for a pre-chemotherapy examination by Drs. Carbone and Charles Loprinzi. I also wore my "Alice in Wonderland" red high-heeled shoes. I bought them in New York just before Dr. Cody diagnosed cancer. I wrapped the boa around me, my makeup was done to perfection, and my hair was smartly done. I sat on the examining table with my legs crossed. When the doctors opened the door and saw me sitting there in my finery, they broke up. "I may have had a mastectomy," I told them, "but I'm still going to be sexy." They took a picture and called in all the doctors and nurses to see the new "gown."

Dr. Carbone wanted to know what I was going to do for the men's gowns. "I'll think of something," I said.

Before my first examination and chemo treatment, I had to sign the necessary papers to be part of this special protocol. But, before I signed the consent forms, I told Drs. Carbone and Loprinzi, who is working on a fellowship under Dr. Carbone, that they had to agree to a few conditions. I knew one of the substances I'd be getting—halotestin—could produce masculine features in females. I told them I'd consent if they agreed to stop this particular medicine if any of the following three things happened to me:

1. I grew a mustache.
2. I grew a beard.
3. I grew balls.

They were so surprised they almost fell off their chairs. But they agreed. We shook hands to seal the bargain. They became aware, for the first time, that they were dealing with a woman whose sexuality, up to this point, has been well-defined. I mentioned to them that I'd already had sex since my surgery. Unlike many people, they knew that losing a breast—or two—has no effect on having sex. Their curiosity led them to ask what I'd felt the first time I had sexual relations when I had only one breast. I told them about the man I was dating, who, a couple of weeks after the surgery, told me he felt it was important for me to have sex before I had too much time to think about the mastectomy. After my holiday visitors left, he and I agreed to try it. I was still a sexy lady. I felt good about it. We had laughter, friendship, and kindness. I told the doctors it was better for the man than for me. They asked if I was going to give up. "Hell no," I said. "I'm just practicing."

The anticipation was far worse than the actual treatment. The only pain came from being there and from the needle. Future experiences with chemo may be worse. But I will not expect the worst. I'll take the treatments one at a time and take whatever comes. Dr. Carbone told me that the side effects of at least one of the drugs might limit my course of treatment. One of the drugs—adriamycin—can adversely affect the heart. I am literally sitting on top of a bomb.

He also told me, "If you are here in a year, we are doing well. If longer, great. If you're not, we didn't do well."

But I'm going to lick this disease. I'm determined to live for more than their estimate of two to five years. I would like to be a wife again. I want to see my children growing older and my grandchildren growing up. I want those moments of laughter. I want to remember that there are beautiful people in the world—a world in which I am living because of my struggle to survive. I want years of sitting under my Purple Tree with its many new branches.

My Purple Tree is my imaginary refuge where I go when I'm depressed. A tree symbolizes growth and peace, it puts out branches that give shade and protection, and it lets you sit underneath and look up at the sky. Purple symbolizes passion and imagination, two facets of my being that combine to give me strength.

January 6, 1984

Am I in pain? Yes. I didn't realize the chemo treatment would be painful. But I will not allow it to take over my life. I discovered last night that a glass of wine took the pain away for a couple of hours.

January 7, 1984

What a nice surprise! Gail, Al's sister, came from the East Coast to visit me during this first week of chemotherapy. She's a nurse and thought she could be of some help to me. Just having her here is a great help. Gail was my room-mate at the Alpha Epsilon Phi sorority house at the University of Wisconsin in Madison. I met her family and was fond of them even before I met Al. She and I are still friends.

I love having Gail here. She's married. She and her husband, a professor at the University of Maryland, live in Columbia, Maryland. They have three children—two boys and a girl. She went back to school in the late 1970s for nurse's training. My former in-laws were very proud of her ambition in getting her degree and going back to work. What a difference 10 years makes! In the sixties I had suggested going back to school for either an MBA or a law degree, and they were aghast.

In 1972, when I opened Catalyst, Inc., the family had some reservations. I have often referred to Catalyst as my third most successful venture. My first was graduating from the University of Wisconsin. My second was my two sons, Marc and Joel. Catalyst, Inc., was the first interior design boutique in Madison when it opened on August 28, 1972. In the shop's 2000 square feet, I showed mostly contemporary designs in leather furniture and avant-garde lighting. There was a gallery where local artisans could show and sell their work as well as a mini art gallery. I introduced exhibition art posters as an art form to Madison. The ambience was informal. For example, on Saturday mornings we had coffee and cake. People could come in to buy or order something, or just to have coffee and talk.

I had four employees. The first person I hired was Susan Engstrom, who has become one of my closest friends. I was only open from 9:30 A.M. to 3 P.M. They said it couldn't be done. I said it *had* to be done because I was going to be home when my boys got home from school.

Al was involved with the business because I recognized that his advertising and public relations skills could help us. For starters, he came up with the name Catalyst. I loved having him involved and I let him know his ideas were appreciated.

Catalyst, Inc. grew.

I remember vividly that, when I started the business, my banker patted me on the shoulder and told me that 90 percent of all small businesses go broke in a year. I patted him on his shoulder and told him I would be in the 10 percent that didn't.

As the business grew I had customers from all over the state. It was succeeding beyond even my wildest dreams. I needed Al's help to franchise it and expand into imports. I had the financial backing. Now I needed my family's support and help. But Al said no. He could not accept my success, nor could he acknowledge that it was also his success. He wanted me to quit work and stay home. He had had it!

I will admit I was exhausted. I had been playing Super Mom/Wife/Businesswoman. I wanted my family—not a divorce. On February 28, 1975, Al and I made a pact: I would give up Catalyst and he would give up his women. I kept my part of the bargain: I gave up my business. He did *not* give up his women. If he had kept his word—and been a mensch— our family would have stayed together. He gave up nothing for his family.

I left my business just as businesswomen were coming into their own as a result of the feminist movement. I was written up—without my knowledge—in *Glamour* magazine. They called me a defeatist because I had "pulled the robes of motherhood around me and gone back to my family." I have never thought of myself as a defeatist. I made a choice and, right or wrong, I've lived with it.

As I reflect on the changes that make Gail's nursing career perfectly acceptable today, I can be almost amused at the final irony. I gave up Catalyst and my career. Now, with cancer and a shortened life expectancy, I probably will not work again. But Al thinks I should have a full-time job! As always, truth is stranger than fiction.

January 9, 1984

Dr. Carbone and his staff warned me I might be depressed during and after the course of treatment. They were right. Today I was terribly depressed. Fortunately I have my great psychologist, Wil Fey, to help me get through these down times. I began consulting Wil in 1980 to help me adjust to the breakup of my marriage.

January 12, 1984

Today I had the second round of the standard chemo protocol. In three weeks I will have the first treatment of what I'm calling the "Big Three"—adriamycin, vinblastine and Thio-tepa.

January 15, 1984

Today I had a reminder of another business in my past. I received an order for my divorce kit. The first year after my 1980 separation was devastating. To help me get through that period I created the kit, *Divorce—A Beginning*. We give gifts to people for every imaginable occasion; why not for the end of a marriage?

Each box contained an address book for new friends, a brochure with advice from professionals for legal, financial, and emotional independence, a poem titled "Divorce," a box of tissues, invitations to a "new beginning" party, napkins and swizzle sticks for the party, announcement cards, and a decision-making flip coin with "laugh" on one side, "cry" on the other.

I'm never without my flip coin. I held on to it through my first appointment with Dr. Cody, and I intend to hold on to it through all my chemotherapy treatments. It's my good luck charm.

January 19, 1984

It's only two weeks since I began chemo and I've already gained 35 pounds. Ugh!

But I had good news from Al's parents, Sam and Ernestine. They know about my illness. They also know my medical bills will be high. They've very generously offered to forgive my monthly mortgage payments to them for an apartment building I bought from Sam in 1975. Ernestine called to tell me their lawyer is working out details. How sweet of them!

January 23, 1984

The phone started ringing early this morning. Several friends called to tell me about an article in the morning paper. It's about an award given in a medical malpractice suit to a woman who had an experience with cancer similar to mine. The only difference—she is dead. I thought: It could be me! Yet, I'm not dead. I've just started the treatments for survival.

I picked up a paper and read the article. Everything came back to me. I'm still not sure how or why this could have happened to me, especially when I was under the care of a doctor I trusted.

Coincidentally, I'm having lunch with Bob Jackson tomorrow. He is back from his vacation in Hawaii and called to say he wanted to know how I am. I agreed to meet him.

January 24, 1984

I met Bob for lunch. I told him I'd had several calls from friends about the lawsuit. He just laughed it off. He was his usual charming self. He talked about how terrible chemotherapy could be and how sure he is I will get through this ordeal in good shape. He changed the subject and told me he's taking his family skiing at Vail. I talked more about chemotherapy and about the fact that in a week I would be going in for my first round of the Big Three. He told me I was courageous. He kept saying he was sorry and that we would get through this together.

His words made no sense. I asked him to explain, but I couldn't understand his response. I had trusted this man with my life. Almost two years ago he assured me I didn't have cancer. Now I'm not sure I *will have* my life. And today, after this whole ordeal, I was having lunch with him and listening to his incredible words.

As we left the restaurant he kissed me goodbye and wished me luck with the chemo next week. I told him to have fun in Vail.

And that's when it hit me: while Bob was going off to ski with his family at a famous Colorado resort, I was going off to the third—very tough—treatment in my chemotherapy procedure. When I got into my car, I actually yelled, "How unfair! How wrong!" At that moment I knew I was going to sue this doctor for medical malpractice. He was not my friend. He didn't do right! I knew that I had to go ahead with this suit—for me, for my family, and for other women.

January 25, 1984

I've thought about almost nothing but the medical malpractice suit since yesterday. I've weighed all the pros and cons. I'm convinced I'm doing the right thing. I'm going to find the best attorney I can to represent me. I might have to go outside of Madison because Bob is so well known and respected in this town. I'm starting today to find the right attorney. I know I'll need lots of luck. My greatest fear is that I might die before the trial begins. I need to get going on this while I'm well enough to help on the case.

February 1, 1984

I go back to the hospital tomorrow for another treatment—the Big Three. I'm sad and frustrated. All I can think of is cancer, death, and dying. I think, "What has happened to me, damn it?!" I want to scream. I want my breast back. I want my thinner body back. I want my health and my other life. I know I cannot go back. I know I can never say I don't have cancer. These thoughts reinforce my decision to sue Bob Jackson.

February 2, 1984

Early this morning and then again at mid-morning I took compazine (an anti-nausea medication) in preparation for today's Big Three. Oddly, it not only makes me drowsy, it also makes me slightly nauseated. Fortunately my good friend Beth Rasmussen drives me to the hospital when I have chemo. I held on to Beth as they injected the drugs into me. Even writing about it now makes me gag. I can even smell the medicine.

I started a new routine today, one that I hope will see me through the chemo treatments. After the chemotherapy we went out for a drink. I tried to eat a little too.

February 17, 1984

I had my first appointment with an attorney today. He is from one of the largest firms in the state, with offices in Milwaukee and Madison. He told me I have a good case if all the facts I had given him are true. I gave him permission to see the records. He said he'd be glad to take the case. I was relieved to know that my instincts were still working despite all the horror I'm living with now. I feel sick and am beginning to lose my beautiful hair. I've also started gaining more weight. I look like a round, sick, balding woman. This is not me. But now that I'm committed to the lawsuit, I must keep my head together and get on with my fight for life. At the same time, I'm going to do my damnedest to correct whatever it was that went wrong beginning in March 1982.

February 24, 1984

It's been 10 weeks since the surgery. I am in Utah with my good friend Kay. This is the ski trip we've been planning for the past six months. It'll be my first time skiing in the West as well as the first time I've been on skis in 20 years. I couldn't let a "little" thing like an operation stop me from taking this long-awaited trip. We'll also visit Sidney in Salt Lake City.

Most of my hair is gone. It started falling out about a week after my first treatment with the Big Three. I wear a hat or scarf most of the time. I have only one strand of hair—and I mean *one*. I have a wig too. But I don't like to wear it—it's too hot, even when the temperature is cold.

February 25, 1984

I went to the top of the highest mountain in Snowbird today. From below, the mountains look like walls. I must be free of walls and barriers. But when I look down I have a different attitude. From the top the scene is magnificent. I see trees, valleys and hills. I see space, a clear run.

March 3, 1984

Last week in Utah did me a lot of good. But right now I feel like crying about the way I look. My hair is gone. I keep reminding myself that the medicines are doing their job. My body is in a horrible state of change. But I'm alive. And—believe it or not—sometimes I feel sexier than when I was well. It makes no sense. Maybe being without hair is erotic, I don't know.

Something else that's funny—losing my hair has been harder on some of my friends than it has been on me. There are some who don't want to be seen with me. I've told them point blank, "If you don't want to be seen with me, that's your problem, not mine. I have more important things to worry about."

My sons have been wonderful, making jokes about my head looking like a billiard ball. I've come to terms with the situation. I regularly shampoo and condition my scalp just as if I had hair.

My scalp is shiny. "Mom, I can see myself on your head," one of my boys said. They pat my head with their hands in a loving manner. I do love it. They're very proud of me. They like to go out with me and watch people react. Most people react with humor. But we understand it's difficult for them. It's taking courage for me to smile and joke. My head is a perfect shape and I'm not ashamed of it. It's me.

Who am I kidding? Losing my hair is horrible. But I've come to feel proud of how I'm handling my baldness. The idea that a woman's crowning glory is her hair is not really true. Her biggest glory is her brain.

March 5, 1984

I had another chemo treatment today. I'm sure the doctors have me pegged as more than a little off-the-wall. Once again I talked about my sexual feelings, about the sexual changes I have and feel. I need to talk about my fears and anxieties. I think they're very happy that my psychologist is taking care of that problem.

I've been trying to tell them, "Guys, this is a physical *and* mental problem. They work together." Sex plays an important part in a cancer patient's life. I still believe that sex is one of my strong links to the well world. I feel normal and well—if only for a moment—during sexual intercourse. I have a great need to be held, touched, and loved. I need to hold on to this part of me that makes me feel good about myself.

With my whole world turned upside down, I've decided that no matter what method of satisfaction works during sex,

I'm going to work on it. I will not give up. I tell myself that I *do* feel. I *will* relax. Sometimes nothing feels good. But my sexuality is definitely part of my feelings about myself and about my worth as a physical, loving woman. Fighting this disease takes so much energy that I often feel I don't have extra energy to expend on sex. But I will *not* give up my ability and need to be intimate. If I've ever needed love, I need it now.

March 7, 1984

Today I received a letter from the Milwaukee attorney telling me he could not take my case because of a conflict of interest. The Jackson Clinic had been a client of his firm. He said it appeared from the reading of the facts in my case that a Jackson Clinic doctor might be involved. (Not Bob. He's not connected with that clinic.) He was sorry. He still believed I had a good case. He was kind enough to recommend three Milwaukee attorneys I might want to contact. I'll have to find out more about these lawyers before I call them.

March 26, 1984

Something new has developed. I call it the "cancer rage." I believe that people who have chemotherapy and radiation get it. I think it's part of living with the fear and frustration of this disease. The drugs lower my blood count, which in turn lowers my resistance. Something happens inside. The drugs seem to control my body. I become picky and nervous. I scream at almost anything or anyone around me when the rage hits. I look the same, but the drugs trigger a change in my feelings, and that changes me. I've been told that the drugs and the side effects are cumulative. So things will probably get worse. But I'm determined to survive, come what may.

March 28, 1984

I called one of the Milwaukee attorneys recommended to me. We met in Madison. He was unsatisfactory: pompous and quite rude. I don't think I'll retain him. I know that if I feel this way about him now, I would not like anything he would do. He wanted to take the case. He emphasized that it wouldn't be easy and would be costly. I told him I wanted to think it over.

April 2, 1984

This was not a good day. I had the second fix of the Big Three. I can hardly keep everything together. I want to cry. I want to quit chemotherapy. When I feel this way, my doctors comment, "You don't have a common cold. You have cancer. You are on some of the most powerful drugs known. Why would you feel good?" Of course they're right. It's an effort to try to feel well. I'm doing my best. I don't want this cancer to move one more step into my life than it already has. At the same time, I never can get away from thinking that I have cancer. "I have cancer" is a phrase that frightens most people. The disease becomes a way of life. It envelops your being, a fact I've finally recognized.

I *am* fighting it. I've said over and over again—especially when I feel down—"I'm going to fight you, you son of a bitch." I've never sworn so much in my life as I have since the diagnosis of cancer. It just happens. I think it's the frustration built into the situation. I want to use obscene words because that's what I think of the disease. Sweet, goody-goody words cannot adequately describe cancer.

April 3, 1984

Thank God for Wil Fey. I felt awful today when I went to see him. I was terribly depressed. I was scared that no one would pick me up. But his office is my security. He helps me feel better—feel good about myself. Wil offers safety and reassurance. He is my umbilical cord to the safe world.

April 23, 1984

The chemo staff gets a kick out of me. They say I'm different from others who receive the same drugs. I refuse to vomit. I refuse to get ill. I want to talk about sex and feelings as part of my treatment. I want them to know how difficult it is being alone, and about the odd, cold feelings in my body. I reminded them today of that great oldie that Fred Waring and his chorus used to sing: "The head bone connected to the neck bone, the neck bone connected to the shoulder bone," and so on. That got a laugh. Humor is essential to getting well. I guess that's why I joke about my illness, my looks, and sex. Laughter is wonderful!

When I say I refuse to throw up, it doesn't mean I am not sick to my stomach. I pick at my food and sometimes I can barely swallow it. I'm constantly nauseated, except when I have a drink. When I drink white wine I feel better. I don't know why. Maybe it's the sugar content, the alcohol, or maybe I'm just more relaxed. There is something in it that helps me. It seems to give me energy and subdue the nausea. I'm sure AA wouldn't like to hear this, but I'm thinking of writing a book titled *How to Get through Chemotherapy with Alcohol*.

April 24, 1984

Feeling good is becoming more difficult with each month on the drugs. Even though I expected that, I felt so lousy today that I called the clinic and said I was going to quit. I wasn't going to take any more of their drugs. "I'm sick of being sick. I'm sick of not having my hair. I'm sick of feeling like shit," I said.

April 25, 1984

Of course I'm not stopping chemotherapy. That was the cancer rage talking. But it did help to get all that frustration and hostility off my chest. I feel more relaxed and calm today.

April 29, 1984

I got on the scale today. I've gained another 20 pounds. I hate being fat. But the doctor tells me that it's not so bad because it enables them to give me more medicine. I'm taking the medicines. At the same time, I can't wait for it to be over. The big red Xs on my calendar mark off each treatment. I don't sleep well. I walk the floors. I'm near panic a lot of the time. And although my heart is crying, I often find it impossible to cry real tears. Part of the problem is the effect chemotherapy has had on my eyes. I've lost my eye lashes; there isn't anything to protect my eyes. They tear and blur, but it's so uncomfortable that I must try not to cry.

May 2, 1984

I've decided not to hire the Milwaukee attorney I talked with a month ago. I had several more contacts with him during the month, and I'm certain now that I do not want him to represent me. I wrote him today telling him of my decision.

I feel rotten and am bald, more in the mood to sue. Bob continues to call to find out how I'm feeling, but I don't take his calls. My head is in the right place now, and I know I was wronged by this doctor. Three times within 20 months he assured me I did not have cancer. I *did* have cancer. I *do* have cancer. And it might very well kill me.

I'm going to find a Madison lawyer. I don't think I'll be wanting to go back and forth to Milwaukee to prepare my case. That would take too much time. And I'm not sure I'll have the energy to do all that traveling. I don't have anyone else to drive me and I don't want to ask the boys to be my chauffeurs.

May 9, 1984

I talked with several local lawyers about Keith Clifford and David Relles who won the malpractice suit publicized in January. They have fine reputations. I interviewed them today, and they interviewed me. I was at their office for two hours. They reiterated what the first attorney said: if I'm telling the truth, I certainly do have a case. They are sincere, warm, and smart.

May 11, 1984

Panic set in yesterday. I thought my lawsuit was ending even before we started. I was ready to hire an attorney to represent me. He asked for, among other things, records of the mammogram and ultrasound test done in New York in December. I had brought them back to Madison with me. Now they were missing. Bob's office said they didn't have them. Then I called the Clinical Cancer Center. They couldn't find them either. Dr. Carbone said he would find them. His office located the records back at Dr. Cody's office in New York. I think Bob's office had sent them back.

On top of that Marc was upset with his job and Joel was worried about finals, which were coming up in a few days.

We decided to have dinner together and cheer each other up. I planned an elegant dinner: crab legs, lobster tails, corn on the cob, artichokes, vegetables, croissants, and wine. With my best china and silver. And candlelight.

During the preparation the oven blew up. Thank God, no one was hurt. What a mess! But we salvaged the lobster tails, and our collective sense of humor was intact.

We were able to joke and laugh as we discussed our various dismal situations. We knew we were all going to make it.

May 16, 1984

I formally hired Clifford and Relles to be my attorneys in my medical malpractice suit against Bob Jackson. I gave them a $1000 retainer and felt secure knowing I had made the right choice. I had decided to look no further. Good men!

May 18, 1984

I guess I should have known it was too good to be true. I found out this morning that there may be a problem with Keith Clifford and David Relles representing me in my suit against Bob Jackson. It seems that he is Mrs. Clifford's doctor. Keith says he's fairly confident, however, that he can work things out. I certainly don't like the idea of having to look for another attorney.

May 21, 1984

Today was Big Three day again. As I sat in the chemotherapy room, I realized that everyone faces death in a different way. All the patients I saw there were fighting this lousy disease. They all need support. I wanted the boys to come with me. They didn't. But they always want me to be up—not easy to do. I have a responsibility—to them and to me—to get well.

Today was like the other chemo days. When I have the injection, I just close my eyes and try to pray the pain away. I really don't want to see the other patients. I want to picture something nice. I use imagery therapy. I'm not really there at all. I hold my hand out and the needle stings me. I hold onto Beth and make small talk and keep thinking I must be brave. I must have the courage to finish this. I tell myself this at the very moment they put the needle into my vein. I'm almost in tears. I feel so sick. I think of my wonderful boys and of my mother. She is a strong woman. If she can do it—survive against all odds—then I can too. We are made of the same stuff.

I noticed today that there's been a change in my voice. I'm calmer, even though the pain is overwhelming at times. I feel like someone is cutting me up inside. I walk holding onto things because my balance is affected. My legs hurt. My skin hurts at the touch. Everything hurts. But on the bright side, I've lived another month. And I've gotten through another chemo series. That's all to the good!

Something else that's good is the friendship I've developed with two of the technicians in the hospital's blood-drawing lab. Lynn Davidson, Pat Vilbrandt, and I have become good friends. I've always hated having blood drawn, but they've drawn mine without my jumping off the chair. The three of us have spent a couple of enjoyable evenings over drinks and dinner.

May 28, 1984

As if the cancer and chemotherapy aren't enough to make life difficult, now I must contend with going back to court with Al tomorrow. I need his help because I have cancer. I asked for his assistance in paying my medical bills. He makes a good salary, so affordability is not the question. When I asked him for some help, I had in mind an agreement that if something should happen to me in the next two years—when my divorce stipulation ends—I will not die with empty pockets. I want to make sure the boys will have something. I still have my business head, even though it's hairless.

Wisconsin law provides that if some unusual circumstance develops during the life of a divorce stipulation, it can be changed. I certainly qualify. I know it's very unlikely, if not impossible, that I'll work again.

I thought we could avoid attorneys' fees if Al and I could agree on an additional amount. I wanted—and hoped to get—

his cooperation. But a leopard doesn't change his spots. He's going to court.

For 22 years the pattern was the same. He was always very nice to me right after he cheated and got caught. What kept me in that marriage for 22 years? I stayed because I didn't have any place to go. I had a baby, then two. Society didn't look as favorably upon single parents then—the 1960s—as it does now. I was not yet trained as an interior designer. My father was dead; Mother couldn't help. So I stuck it out, hoping it would get better. I had expected some hard times. I felt abused. And sometimes I felt that it was my fault. I didn't know I was feeling like the classic battered wife.

In spite of all my problems with this man, both during our marriage and since the divorce, I can still say we were a good pair. I did love him. We were creative and—when he wasn't with another woman—we had a good marriage. At those times he was caring and wanted to make the marriage work. Then suddenly—without warning—the fighting would start. I knew that meant he was seeing another woman. In my opinion, in order for him to succeed with another woman, he had to see me as a bitch. I fought back. I guess that made me his bitch.

On July 5, 1979, our 20th anniversary, he promised he would not have any more affairs if I would take him back. He said he wanted to make himself worthy of me and be a good husband. I warned him that if he had one more affair I would divorce him. This was his last chance.

He promised. I said, "If you think you can't do this, let's get help. I will help you."

We had a wonderful six weeks. In September it ended. He took up with another person. This time I was finished. He lied to the very end. Until April 17, 1980, he denied he was having an affair. On that day a minor miracle happened. An anonymous female caller told me where Al's current love letters were hidden. Her information was accurate.

I believe the stress of my marriage and my separation and divorce in 1980 were contributing factors in causing my cancer. I believe the stress threw my system out of balance.

May 29, 1984

I spent part of the day in court. I was so nervous that I broke out in hives all over my body. It wasn't easy to sit there listening to Al talk. The attorneys spent what seemed like hours going over budgets. How much for chemotherapy? How much for counseling? What amount of food do I eat? How much do our sons eat? All this was costing $100 an hour.

Finally I interrupted and told the court commissioner that I really didn't concentrate on my expenses. I explained that I don't even know if I will live this year out. I'm only worried now about getting through chemotherapy. I mentioned that I go out to dinner a lot because cooking and eating at home is difficult. I showed him letters from my doctors stating that I can't work at this time. I ended with, "If I had my way, I would not be dependent on this man for the rest of my life. All I really want is to live and be well."

The commissioner ordered Al to pay more. I was exhausted. The stress was incredible. But I won. If I cannot care for myself at home and need professional help, Al will have to pay my bills.

I feel liberated, and sad. The boys did not want Al to take me to court. They told me they've lost what little respect they had for him.

June 1, 1984

While waiting to see Dr. Carbone today I started talking with another patient. He was bald and had radiation markings on his head. He was with his wife, whom I knew from the time my mother was in the hospital three years ago. I said, "Your bald head looks terrific. It takes one to know one." With that, I unwrapped the scarf from my head and told him that I am on chemotherapy. We got into a discussion of our feelings about having cancer. He said that losing his beautiful beard and mustache was more difficult than losing his hair. We talked more about our feelings and promised that if either of us wanted to talk we would call.

I'm not afraid to go up to people and talk. I learn from people. I'm a people watcher.

Dr. Carbone said today that he feels some of my depression is due to the fact that I'm doing this alone. He's right. Being alone with cancer gets to me. I have my mom and my boys, but I miss having a special man to be close to. Loneliness can creep up on you. You really have to push out to avoid it. Being alone is one thing; being lonely is something else.

Here is where I retreat and go to sit under my Purple Tree. There I have time to reflect and look out at the world from beneath its sheltering branches. I can laugh. I can understand that something positive can come out of something bad. I create my own happiness by always ending the day with a positive thought. I'm alive! And my new life is about living the best way I know how. I have adopted a new motto: I do only what I feel good about. I can't waste my limited energy on anything else.

Writing these thoughts in this journal has brought back a lot of memories, memories that seem to explain me and my reaction to this terrible disease that has invaded my life. I was really quite young—12 to be exact—when I realized I saw people and things around me in a different way. I felt like an adult, although I was still a child. (I know there are some people who think I act like a child now that I am an adult.) I used to listen to my father and his friends talk business. I found their discussions interesting. I was fascinated by their thinking, their words, and their anger and eventual agreement on controversial subjects. I'm sure no one thought I could even understand their conversations. I knew, though, that I wanted to be like them. Although I was only 14, I got a job in the window shade department of a dime store. I was getting paid two dollars an hour and I thought it was fabulous. The following year I went to work for a department store in Chicago. I was still underage, but I was experienced.

Next I got a job at an ice cream parlor. But I wanted to know more about merchandising. So at age 15½ I applied at the two best stores in town—Bonwit Teller and Bramson's. Both said they didn't hire people under 16. Every two months I went back to ask how close I was to being hired. On my 16th birthday Bramson's personnel manager said, "You can sell yourself, you can sell our clothes." That same afternoon Bonwit's called. That's when I first realized that perseverance pays. I knew I could get what I wanted if I didn't get discouraged and give up. I took the job at Bramson's in Evanston. Leo Bramson was a good merchandiser. He taught me buying, window display, fashion coordination, salesmanship, management—all aspects of retailing. I even helped with their radio program that aired Saturdays at Northwestern University.

I believe the determination that got a younger Diane the job she wanted is going to see the older Diane through this rotten time in her life.

June 6, 1984

I had my first date with Kurt last night. He is a widower, about 20 years older than I am. He is also bald. He made dinner for us. He is an excellent cook.

June 9, 1984

Kurt left today for a three-week vacation in Europe. In two days I begin another round of chemotherapy.

I'm still trying to get Marc and Joel to go with me for a treatment. So far they've been reluctant to do so. I've told them repeatedly, "I'm the one with the illness. I'm the one who's taking this poison. How can you know what I'm going through if you don't see what they're doing to me?" I was sick—I went through the rage—and they still would not go. I want them to feel what I am feeling, even though I know that's not possible. They have their own feelings. I guess it's true that when you're young, you think you're going to live forever. And they probably think I will too, that this part of my life is some sort of aberration in which they have no parts to play.

July 8, 1984

Sidney has been visiting from Salt Lake City. This afternoon she and I went downtown to the Art Fair on the Square. I discovered a fine young leather artist who was one of the exhibitors. I was impressed with the style and artistic flair of her pieces. I commissioned her to make an outfit—in rust and red leather—of wrapped skirt, poncho, and beret.

July 10, 1984

I seem to have been going nonstop for the past 24 hours. Kurt returned from Europe yesterday. We had dinner at his house, and I stayed the night.

July 25, 1984

Mom and I had dinner at a Mexican restaurant last night. Just the two of us. I'm completely bald. It's too hot to wear anything on my head. I could tell Mom was a little uncomfortable about my baldness. While we were eating, a woman came to the table and took my hand. She said she'd been "there" a year ago. She began crying. She had breast cancer too. She assured me that it does get better. I wanted to kiss her. She said, "Good for you. You're not wearing a wig. I took mine off one day to go to the grocery store and never wore it again."

I told her I stopped wearing the wig because it was too hot. But the real reason was that I couldn't figure out how to make love holding on to my head!

I needed that pep talk. And—coming from a total stranger—it helped even more than had it come from a friend or doctor. I am, frankly, a mess. I look like a skinned chicken. I have hot flashes caused by Tamoxifen. It intercepts estrogen on its way to receptive cells in my breast. I worry about infection because the drugs lower my resistance. My pubic hair is gone and the lips of my labia rub on my underpants, which I must change several times a day. I also have a disagreeable and uncomfortable vaginal discharge. The exhaustion is overwhelming. It never leaves me. Nor does the depression. Sometimes I'm ready to scream at the unfairness of it all. I didn't know it was possible to feel this lousy and continue with the business of daily life.

July 26, 1984

I don't know what set me off. Perhaps it was the reminder when I looked at the calendar yesterday that I go for another round with chemotherapy beginning August 2, one week from today. But this morning I woke up screaming for help. A sudden wave of cancer, death, depression, and pain came over me. I felt so alone. I asked God to hear me and help. I didn't know how I was even going to get out of bed, much less get through the day. I felt paralyzed, literally unable to move. This was not the first time the cancer rage had taken over. I was ready to explode quite often. I've tried to tell those I love about it. Marc and Joel, as well as some of my friends, have finally admitted the cancer rage is not a figment of my imagination. They recognize it, but no one can keep it at bay.

This episode was one of the worst and one of the most unusual because the rage erupted before chemotherapy rather than after. The rage itself follows the same pattern every time. I fall into a depression that drowns me like a tidal wave. Then I imagine I have one tiny hole to swim through to get out of this wave of darkness, to get back to the land and under my Purple Tree. I imagine myself lying under the tree, looking at the sky, and putting my body in a weightless state. Even with my faith and imagery I know I will never completely regain a healthy me. But I have the will to fight, and that's half the battle. When I get up I have the strength to carry on. I go about my normal routine: take a bath, brew a pot of coffee, put on a favorite recording, dress, and put on my makeup. I don't have to do my hair! I look the best I can. And, thank God, I can also see and talk with my psychologist.

August 17, 1984

Kurt and I are in New York. I came back to see Dr. Cody. Although he tells me I have some of the best medical care in the world at the UW Hospital and Clinical Cancer Center, I keep coming back. After all, he did save my life. And I do love New York. We're staying with Felice and Harry.

I had an amusing encounter this afternoon at the Museum of Modern Art. A woman in her early twenties came up to me and said it was nice to see a middle-aged woman so modern and so punk with an avant-garde hairdo. "Good for you," she said. "Keep going, lady. Love your 'do'." Then she turned and walked away. I wanted to tell her that with a year of chemotherapy and for about $20,000 she too could be bald.

August 20, 1984

I saw Dr. Cody earlier today. He told me I am doing very well and that he's proud of my acceptance of chemotherapy. He added, "They are doing everything right. You have a chance."

Then he told me something pretty scary and—I hope—not prophetic. He said, "Don't be concerned about finding a lump in your breast. If it's going to come back, it will be on the right side, in exactly the same place as the first one." Then he showed me where it could recur. *In exactly the same place as the first one.*

After that report, I went out and bought myself another goody. That's part of every trip to New York; when I get a good report, I splurge and buy myself a nice present.

Then—to carry on with this ritual—Felice and I went out for a drink. We paid $12 for two strawberry daiquiris at a midtown bar! But who cares about the price? What's important is that I am here and able to have a drink with a friend. We met Kurt and Harry for our usual celebratory dinner. Then we went to a Broadway show. We saw the British production *Noises Off*. Very good.

August 30, 1984

I don't think I'm what the Scots call "fey." I don't have true second sight and I'm not clairvoyant. But I believe I am able to foresee some events. I guess I'd say I get vibes, and they've never failed me. This morning I have my next date with the Big Three, and I am petrified. All day yesterday I had bad vibes. I went out to dinner last night with my good friend Linda. I told her I was scared. I didn't think it would go well today. I just had this feeling that nothing was going to go right. She felt helpless, but she did try to calm my fears.

For the first time the boys are coming to the hospital with me. As usual, Beth will drive me there and stay with me during the treatment. I'm glad they're all coming. I need their support. I hope what I've been feeling is someone else's bad dream.

August 31, 1984

Yesterday was not someone else's bad dream. It was my own very real nightmare, more terrifying than an Alfred Hitchcock movie.

Things went wrong from the beginning. For the first time since I started chemotherapy my blood count was too low for me to have a treatment. I had a choice: either come back in a few days or go down to the cafeteria, eat as much protein and sweets as I could in 30 minutes, then walk around the hospital and come back. They would then draw blood again and test it. I chose the second option; as long as I was there I wanted to get it over with. I ate what I could. Then I took off my high-heeled shoes and, since I wasn't wearing stockings, walked around the hospital barefooted for about 15 minutes. The second time around my blood count was at an acceptable level.

Before the treatment Sandy gave me a shot to help me relax and to kill the pain. I knew the treatment would be painful, so I had asked for the shot. Sandy knew it too.

Then we proceeded. Sandy was in charge. She gave all the medications as prescribed by the doctor and prepared in the clinic pharmacy. When we finally got to the last and most difficult medicine—adriamycin—it burned. I told Sandy I was cold and was having a tough time breathing. It felt like an elephant was on my chest. I knew Sandy was alarmed. I saw it in her eyes. She called to another nurse to stay with me. As she ran out of the room, she yelled over her shoulder, "I'm getting Charlie."

Fortunately I was already lying down on one of the treatment room's recliners. The pre-treatment shot had made me too tired to sit in my usual chair. At this point, I couldn't have sat up anyway. My vein—where the medicines were injected—was inflamed. Although mine was not a code blue emergency, they were ready to take very quick action if things got worse.

The medication was done. Charlie decided to keep a close watch on me. The boys' eyes reflected the seriousness of the situation. However, Sandy knew I was stabilizing. She said, "If the pendulum was going to swing toward a drastic, acute reaction, I would know by now."

Although the crisis was past, I was alternately chilled and sweaty as the medication started to take effect. They gave me a shot of Benedryl. I almost doubled over. I felt like a knife was cutting into my stomach. One nurse was holding my hand while Sandy took my vital signs. They put more blankets over me. The boys were watching all this. They were stunned. Sandy suggested that they and Beth leave for a few minutes, but Joel wouldn't leave. He stayed, holding onto the big toe on my right foot. He kept asking if I was okay and never let go of my toe. A nurse stayed with me the whole time too. Marc and Beth returned about 15 minutes later. I finally started to come around and they agreed to let me go home. The boys assured the staff that I would not be alone. They promised that if anything went wrong they would bring me to the emergency room immediately.

At that point I did not have the time, energy, or control to figure out what had happened. But, I thought, I've had it with adriamycin. Sandy told me that she had always felt there was the possibility something might go wrong during one of my treatments. Good thing I didn't know that when chemo started: I might never have gone through it.

This incident was a real eye-opener for the boys. They'd always thought Mom was just going for her chemotherapy, that it was like any other shot. But yesterday's episode shook them up. They had an unforgettable lesson. Chemotherapy was wicked to them too. As it turned out, they took care of me. They were in charge and did a wonderful job. I felt comforted and secure with them. Mom came over too. I wanted her with me. She gave me added strength.

But my miserable day wasn't over. I had another incident of cancer rage after Mom got here, and she took the brunt of it. She and the boys ordered Chinese food for dinner. I was in bed. I needed complete rest. She came in to check on me and I suddenly started up about how she ought to go back to school and learn more about the Civil War. It's a subject she's interested in. I got out of bed and went to look for my Civil War books by Bruce Catton. I couldn't find them in the den. It was a mess. So I took out some other books for her to read. She finally got me back to bed and left the room. I laughed and cried at the same time. I was hysterical. I guess I didn't know what I was doing. I was a raging, crazy lady for a few minutes. After a while I settled down. I still can't believe it had happened so fast.

Now I know that the rage is chemically produced. It's real and it's frightening. But it does pass. Last evening's episode reaffirmed my belief that many oncology patients would benefit from psychological or psychiatric help to get them through chemotherapy and the rage, whatever form it takes. It's a terrifying experience for those who go through it and for those around them.

Last night Marc helped me calm down too. Now he has seen exactly what chemotherapy is all about. But I'm still alone with cancer. Thank God Marc and Joel don't share my world. I know it was tough for them. But in the past 24 hours I believe the boys have finally understood just what I'm going through. I'm more grateful than I can ever say for their love and patience. They're doing their very best, even though it's impossible for them to imagine what happens inside the body of a person who is on chemotherapy.

If I live, cancer may be one of the best things that ever happened to me. That's a strange thing to say, but I have done more in these months—while I've had every reason not to do anything—than I would have done otherwise. I don't feel sorry for myself, most of the time. Cancer has made me realize that living can only be done on a day-to-day basis.

September 1, 1984

Even Kurt was alarmed at the events of the last two days. He bought a television set for my bedroom because he knew I was sick and needed to stay in bed for a few days.

I was right about the adriamycin. Apparently I'm allergic to it. Once this medicine gets into my body, it simply accumulates until I have a reaction like the one I experienced two days ago. I called my Uncle George, the anesthesiologist in Florida, about this turn of events. (Uncle George and Aunt Nish Finer are really Al's relatives. Their support, love, and advice have sustained me for 26 years.) He said I must stop taking this drug. One more treatment would not necessarily make a big difference in my life. I called Dr. Cody. He was alarmed, but told me to do exactly what my doctors here advised. I also called one of the top physicians in the UW Hospital cardiac department, someone I know. He too advised against continuing. He said it could damage my heart and it could be fatal.

Sandy Larson called to check on me and to tell me the doctors are studying the situation. They are weighing all the pros and cons involved in continuing adriamycin. She said Dr. Carbone would call me when they've decided what course to take.

September 5, 1984

Much against everyone's better judgment—mine included—I'm leaving later today for Columbia, Maryland. My niece, Gail's daughter, will have her Bat Mitzvah on Saturday. I'm still very ill and very shaken after the events of last Thursday. But Jamie is a sweet girl. She is very special to me.

September 15, 1984

Although I'm nearing the end of chemotherapy, I still need to rest a lot. The drugs and their side effects are cumulative. I continue to be amazed at how completely the drugs take control. My mood swings are unpredictable. They shock me. One minute I'm happy and calm, the next depressed and agitated. I may resemble myself, but I am not me.

That's one reason I've started exercising regularly at the University of Wisconsin Sports Medicine and Fitness Center. Darryl Miller and Jackie Kuta, two staff exercise physiologists, have been especially supportive. They've tailored a program for me. They know my limitations and they encourage me whenever I'm there. Regardless of how I feel, I want to look good again.

September 26, 1984

Yesterday was an extraordinary day in my life. It didn't begin that way. When Kurt and I left to attend the funeral of his cousin in Chicago, I had no idea of what lay ahead. The funeral was at Westlawn Cemetery, where my father is buried.

I hadn't been back to his grave for seven or eight years. I thought I remembered where Dad's grave was, and as we drove into the cemetery I suddenly wanted very much to find it. As we got out of the car I saw the rabbi who was to officiate at the funeral. It was Rabbi Schulman—the same man who had married Al and me 25 years ago! I introduced myself; he remembered our wedding. We chatted for a few moments about the years since then.

There was an eerie sensation about this whole place and the coincidence of meeting Rabbi Schulman. I began to feel extremely vulnerable. Being there revived old thoughts about how much I missed Dad. I have often thought, when depression hits hard, that the bad things in my life started with his death. He was my best friend.

As I joined in the Kaddish, the prayer for the dead in the funeral service, I began to feel as if it was my funeral, as if I had died and was lying under the stone. I knew I wasn't dead, but I started crying and couldn't stop the tears. Then, as suddenly as this weird feeling came over me, it vanished. I realized, I am alive! This was not my funeral. I thought, God, I'm not ready for this, I've got a lot of living to do.

After the service I looked for Dad's grave but couldn't find it. I went to the cemetery office for directions. I had actually been quite close, but the area had changed so since my last visit that I didn't recognize it. As I stood beside Dad's grave I felt I was with him. I talked to him, as I have every day since his death. I told him he couldn't have me yet, that I'm not ready. I told him not to fight to get me but to fight instead for me to live with my sons, the grandchildren he never knew. I added that I didn't want to leave Mom either. Somehow, I felt, he heard me.

I said goodbye with a prayer and threw a kiss. I wish he hadn't died and left me with so much responsibility. But I felt less alone after being with him for those few minutes. I believe he understood I wouldn't be joining him now. For that matter, I don't intend doing so for a long time. Kurt and I drove back to Madison after visiting with his cousin's family for a short time. The odd feelings I experienced disappeared as mysteriously as they appeared. But it's a day I'll never forget.

September 27, 1984

Hallelujah! My final treatment with the standard protocol is this morning. After that, I'll only be required to take two kinds of pills until the middle of November. No more injections! I can hardly believe it.

September 28, 1984

The last 24 hours have been so busy—and so happy—that I haven't had time to think about my problems. After my last chemo treatment, George Bush took me for a plane ride. He has been a pilot for many years and thought this would be a good way to celebrate my big day. He took me up to his world in the sky, and I loved it. I was sorry we had to come back to earth.

October 1, 1984

No more injections! What a relief. Dr. Carbone made the decision—with my concurrence—to stop adriamycin. The only medications I'll be taking are in pill form—Tamoxifen and Halotestin—until the middle of November. I held my doctors to their agreement—that they cut the dosage of Halotestin if I begin to display masculine features. More facial hair appeared last month. They cut the dosage in half.

I talked with Keith Clifford and David Relles today about what, if any, progress they are making on my malpractice suit. They assured me that things look good. We should be ready to file suit shortly after the first of the year.

October 8, 1984

I had an unexpected encounter this afternoon. Kurt and I were pulling out of the parking lot of a west side shopping mall, and who should be there but Bob Jackson? I introduced him to Kurt. We talked a little about chemotherapy and the fact that I have no hair.

He told me I looked good.

I told him, "I'm going to sue you. Something has to be done for me."

He answered that if I wanted to sue him, I would have to sue the "other guys too."

October 15, 1984

Only one more appointment to keep for chemotherapy: on Thursday. I know I've had 10 months to get used to having only one breast. But I still have mixed feelings about it. On one hand, I had two for the first 46 years of my life. I liked having them around. They were a part of me. On the other hand, I realize that a breast is just one of the appendages of my body. And, somehow, it's not very important. It's not the breast that makes me sexy, even if we do live in a world of two boobs. It's the image of myself, my personality, and my creativity that make the difference. I feel lucky to be alive.

I cannot end this course of chemotherapy without noting and applauding the first-rate medical treatment I've received at the University of Wisconsin Clinical Cancer Center. I'm extremely fortunate to have this world-class facility here in Madison. But it's been difficult to get some of the doctors and nurses to discuss the problem of sexuality during treatment. Despite their reluctance to talk with me about this subject, I still had to deal with the soreness from the loss of my pubic hair, the loss of feeling in my hands and legs, and, more important, the pain and depression that I needed help with. As I've said so many times: Thank God for Wil Fey.

I know that Sloan-Kettering in New York, with Dr. Jimmie Holland, is one of the few places where psychologists and psychiatrists work with cancer patients from the time their illness is diagnosed. We all need this tender, loving care. We need people to say, "It's okay to have these concerns and fears. Now what are we going to do about the seeking of sexual contact and the actual performance?"

I'm speaking here for many men and women who may hesitate to ask questions about sex and sexuality during this trying time in their lives. I'm lucky that my sexuality is intact. My fight against being destroyed during my marriage taught me survival skills, the same skills I am using to fight this rotten disease.

October 18, 1984

This is a red-letter day. At the hospital today I'll have an examination—complete with boa and my exotic red and gold feather headdress—and get what I hope will be the last prescription for my pills. Tonight I'm having an end-of-chemotherapy party at an area restaurant. I think I'll wear the headdress tonight too.

October 19, 1984

In a pre-party mood, I went to the beauty shop yesterday for the first time since February. I have some fuzz on my head and I wanted it colored just like it was before. My good friend Tom Welch did a great job. I told him I couldn't stand for the color to be anything except blonde. When he finished, I had a golden blonde scalp. I have decided I'll go back to him every two weeks while my hair is growing out.

Kurt will have to drop his best one-liner. He's been telling people for months that he and I have the same barber, only he's got more hair than I do.

October 25, 1984

Last night I attended the first session of I Can Cope, a cancer support group at St. Mary's Hospital. I had started this course last spring, but didn't complete it. This time around I'll take the whole eight-week course. Listening to other cancer patients talk at these meetings helps me and the others learn to say the words "I have cancer."

November 1, 1984

I've joked a lot about being bald. It didn't make sense to cry about it or ignore it. It was a fact. I had to live with it. So I tried to make light of it. Now that my hair has started growing back, I'm puzzled. It's coming in curly and dark and looks just like pubic hair. My pubic hair has started growing back too, only it's coming in straight. I thought, "My God, I think the medicines screwed me up completely. I'm upside down!"

November 3, 1984

Kurt asked me to marry him. I said yes. We'll set the date on November 16 when I get back from Salt Lake City.

November 8, 1984

I leave this afternoon for Salt Lake City. I'm going alone. I'll visit Sidney and go up to my beloved mountains. I need this time alone. I must think through the decision to marry Kurt.

November 16, 1984

I got home yesterday. The week away did me a world of good. I told Kurt that I want to wait six months—until April—to get married. I want to have a full head of hair on my wedding day. I'm still sick from the chemotherapy. I need at least that much time for the drugs to work their way out of my system. I still feel like a junkie. Kurt agreed, reluctantly.

I've discussed this matter with my doctors and with Sandy Larson. They all agree: I should not rush into marriage or make any other big decisions that will substantially change my life. I have been a very sick woman. I must give myself time to heal.

November 18, 1984

Today's appointment at the Cancer Center was my last chemo visit. Although I had no treatment, just being there brought back the smell, the pain, and the feeling of total exhaustion I've had for the past 10 months. I want this ordeal to end. I need to leave it behind me.

The doctors are taking me off everything, even the Tamoxifen, which many women continue taking after chemo treatments end. I am ambivalent about this turn of events. One part of me is happy, another part is scared. My security blanket has been taken away. Unconsciously I've built up a sense of trust and confidence in the chemotherapy since January. It's been my friend, not my enemy. And I trust these people. They are dedicated to keeping me alive. After my experience with Bob Jackson, I was not sure I could ever trust a doctor again. But this is a far different place and a far different group of doctors.

I'm excited to think I might get thin again and start feeling well, whatever that might mean. Better than that, I think the side effects will begin to diminish and I'll start thinking clearly again. I can't wait to start a new life without drugs! I'm even looking forward to having a period again. The Tamoxifen causes menopausal-like symptoms.

There is, however, a dark side to these feelings of hope and new beginnings. There is no way of knowing: Has the chemotherapy wiped out the malignancy? Will there ever be a recurrence? My feelings of abandonment and desolation are much like those I had when my father died and, again, when my husband left.

Right now I would welcome having someone assure me that everything will be all right, to take over all of my responsibilities. I know that's unrealistic, that even under my Purple Tree I will not find such a perfect state. I feel like a teenager who has just received her driver's license: loving the freedom of driving, yet feeling the burden of knowing all judgment and responsibility are on her shoulders alone. The hope remains that someone or something is watching over me.

I guess I'll never truly be free from the terror of those words I heard almost a year ago: "Diane, you have breast cancer."

CHAPTER 4

November 19, 1984

Kurt and I met with our attorney today to work out a pre-nuptial agreement. Afterwards we had an argument. We've had them before, and they do not bode well for our marriage.

November 22, 1984

I had my blonde fuzz done specially yesterday for Mom's 75th birthday party at my house. We had about 25 people—family and friends—here to celebrate at a buffet dinner. Mother was in good form. We all had a great time. It's nice to feel like giving a party again.

December 2, 1984

Another setback. Keith and Dave called today to tell me they must withdraw from the case. Since Keith's wife is Bob Jackson's patient, they feel there's too much of a conflict of interest to overcome. They will not put my case in jeopardy by trying to ignore that obstacle. I've been feeling very good about their handling of the case—they were doing a great job. But they didn't leave me up the creek without a paddle, so to speak. They recommended that I talk with Bill Smoler, another young Madison lawyer. They're convinced I have a marvelous case and that I must pursue it.

I called Bill this afternoon. I have an appointment with him tomorrow afternoon.

December 3, 1984

Well that was easier than I expected. I spent several hours with Bill Smoler this afternoon. He's very bright and charming. He's eager to take this case and to win. I think he can do it for me. I formally hired him to represent me. I think we'll get along well.

December 6, 1984

Kurt and I flew to New York yesterday for my appointment with Dr. Cody. I'll see him on Monday.

December 10, 1984

I had a good report after my checkup with Dr. Cody today. He also gave me some good advice. He told me, emphatically, not to make any big decisions about my life, such as getting married. He wants me to give myself "time to get my body back, to relax."

He repeated something he had said many times, that I have wonderful doctors taking care of me. He agreed to talk to Bill and told me when he should call.

December 17, 1984

I had my last appointment with Wil today. He's retiring. He's not leaving me out in the cold, though. He knew I would need a new therapist and did some scouting for me. He suggested that I talk with Fred Coleman, a psychiatrist here in Madison. I've heard good things about him from several doctors and nurses. I'll call his office to make an appointment for after the first of the year.

December 20, 1984

I realized today that I have had another security blanket in addition to the chemotherapy: my leather outfit. I've worn the outfit at least five out of every seven days since I got it. It's the only stylish, classy outfit I own that hides my cancer figure and still makes me look sensuous. To me it represents a link to my world of interior design and a contrast to my world of cancer and chemicals. Wearing this outfit is my artistic way of fighting the disease. It helps me feel confident about winning my fight for life. It's original and creative.

December 23, 1984

I haven't been completely idle during the dark days of this past year. A local jewelry designer and I have created a pin, and I'll have several dozen made. I plan to give them to people who were special to me during the past year.

December 27, 1984

I love Christmas. But for the second straight year Christmas has been a stressful period for me. Last year I had just come home from the hospital and was recuperating from the mastectomy. I was reconciling myself to the shock of having cancer and fearful about the chemotherapy treatments I faced. This year Kurt and I fought about everything.

January 2, 1985

Another New Year off to a sensational start! Kurt has left. Between Christmas and New Year's Day I finally made up my mind: I could not marry this man. Completely aside from the rather precarious state of my health, there were other considerations. We disagreed about almost everything—including my decision to sue Bob Jackson. He didn't want me to pursue the suit. He said he'd take care of me. He was angry with me because I had decided I would never give up this suit. He didn't realize I'm suing for my sanity, not the money. It's a moral issue too. I'm fighting so that others can benefit from my ordeal.

January 7, 1985

Bill Smoler called today. He's just back from a vacation in Spain and the Canary Islands. He told me he'd taken along a suitcase full of medical books and publications. He read them as he sat on the beach. Now he needs to find an expert witness to testify for me at the malpractice hearing. He's planning to call Keith and Dave for any leads they might be able to give him.

January 10, 1985

I called Wil today to let him know I've made an appointment with Fred Coleman, the psychiatrist he suggested I see. I also told him that Kurt and I are no longer together.

January 30, 1985

It's been nice to have the house to myself since Kurt left. I've spent a lot of time conferring with Bill about the malpractice suit. We've gotten to know each other quite well. I know he'll do a good job for me. I have a feeling we'll win this case, even if, as he told me, I might have only a two percent chance of winning. I've been having good vibes about the suit and Bill.

Something else good happened to me today. I had my first appointment with Fred Coleman. What a charming, sympathetic man. We hit it off right from the start. I must call Wil and thank him for sending me to this man for therapy.

February 9, 1985

Mom and I went out for lunch today. Nothing fancy, hot dogs and sauerkraut at a small place we like on the east side. It was snowing when we started home. As we drove, my sense of the ridiculous took over and I said, "Can you believe it? You have the number-one killer disease—heart disease; and I have the number-two killer disease—cancer. Medical science has kept us alive, and we'll probably be killed in this damned car on the highway."

February 11, 1985

I hated doing it, but I had to go back to Al and ask for more money to pay my medical expenses. I didn't want to go back to court. My attorney, Howie Goldberg, handled the request in a letter. Al only had to write a letter consenting to our request. He refused.

The court commissioner was most understanding. Al mentioned the money I lost on the divorce kit. The commissioner asked if I had anything from it. I answered, "Yes. Seven hundred divorce kits in my basement." Everyone laughed.

The commissioner ordered Al to continue his support and to pay half of my psychiatrist's bill.

February 22, 1985

I was at the airport early this morning to leave on a ski trip, made possible by a special Christmas gift.

I couldn't believe it: of all the people to run into, I had to meet Bob Jackson. He was his same charming self, acted as if he had played no part in my ordeal. He came over, kissed me, and asked how I was. I tried to be pleasant, but all I could think about was the turn my life had taken in December of 1983. His cordiality just made me angry. To make matters worse, we were on the same plane to Colorado. I'm determined not to let my encounter with Bob Jackson spoil my trip.

March 8, 1985

The ski trip did me a lot of good. But today, again, I'm not feeling too well. I saw Fred today. I kept saying "there's something wrong." I told him I thought I had cancer again.

March 13, 1985

I've been feeling pretty well for the last few days. But I must have picked up a flu bug. Last night I went out to dinner. When I got home, I felt ill. About three this morning I threw up. It helped, and I finally got some sleep. Of course, in the back of my mind was the thought that all this was caused by cancer. But I feel much better today. I even managed to play a little tennis.

March 28, 1985

I don't feel well today. I'm scared. Things are just not right. I fear there is something dreadfully wrong with me.

But there was good news. Bill called to tell me that he will file the papers for my lawsuit tomorrow, three years to the day that I first went to see Bob Jackson about the lump in my breast.

April 17, 1985

If I had known what was going to happen to me yesterday when I got out of bed, I would have pulled the covers back up and stayed put.

To begin the day I found another lump, exactly where Dr. Cody told me there could be a recurrence. I didn't know whether this was some colossal joke or not. But the discovery was every bit as devastating as finding the first lump. I could not believe that just five months after chemotherapy ended I had that bastard cancer again. And I was sure it was malignant.

Later in the morning, during my appointment with Fred, I said, "I have cancer again. I found a lump." I told him that I was thinking of going out of town for a few days and that I'd do something about the lump when I come back. "It won't make any difference," I said.

Fred didn't try to force any opinion on me. He told me he knew I would make the right decision on my own. As I was leaving, I repeated, "I probably won't do anything about it now." His parting words were, "You'll make the right decision."

I stopped at the stop sign as I drove out of the parking lot. It was decision time. If I turned right, I would go home. If I turned left, I would go to the hospital. I turned left, for three very good reasons. First, my brain was still functioning and I knew I needed help immediately; second, with the lawsuit pending, I would be at fault if I waited; and third, if I did nothing, I might not be alive by the time my suit is heard.

When I got to the hospital I walked into Dr. Pellett's office and told his nurse, "I have cancer again. I want to see Dr. Pellett right now." She told me he would see me as soon as he was free.

Things moved very fast when I did see him. He confirmed the existence of another lump. He asked if I wanted it removed right away or in a day or two. I said, "Right now!"

Pellett did the surgery in an outpatient operating room right there in his department. I had a local anesthetic. By the time I was ready for surgery both George Bush and my good friend Bette, a nurse practitioner, were with me. John Pellett had called them. Each held one of my hands during the surgery. Dr. Pellett sent the excised tumor to the pathology lab. In a very short time the report came back that it was indeed malignant.

At that point he called in the rest of the troops: Dr. Carbone, Dr. Loprinzi, and Sandy Larson. I asked them to call Joel. I wanted him here with me. They finally ran him down at the Nielsen Tennis Stadium across the street from the hospital. He came over right away. I cried in his arms. The nurses left us alone for a few minutes. Then Sandy came in. She watched us and saw the support and strength I drew from his presence. Sandy put her arms around both of us and said, "It doesn't look great. It's not good. But we'll find a way to help."

Damn. Damn! I have cancer again. No one seems to have any answers when I ask *why* this happened. I have to fight again for my life. I would really like to know what makes *me* so special that I should have to wage this battle so soon again. They told me that I will need 30 radiation treatments. But I know I will not be alone. I have God, I have my boys, I have my mom, and some very special friends.

I've cried endlessly today. Now I must dry my tears and get on with the business of survival, again.

April 18, 1985

I had a general checkup and a chest X-ray at the hospital today. I also started taking Tamoxifen again. Five months without it was not good. The tumor was estrogen-positive. Charlie Loprinzi tells me I will be on the Tamoxifen for the rest of my life. He said it could work wonders and that I'll just have to learn to live with the side effects. I *do* feel more secure taking it.

April 19, 1985

I visited the radiation therapy department for the first time today. They made a plaster cast of my upper body. I will lie in the mold for every radiation session to make sure I am in the right place on the table and that I don't move around. Then they drew special colored markings on my chest as guides for the radiation therapists. I told the nurse who painted the pattern to please mark an arrow on my stomach pointing to my crotch. Just in case one needs directions. She did it for me. But she was laughing so hard that the line isn't quite straight.

April 23, 1985

I saw Dr. Pellett today. He checked last week's surgery. Tomorrow I begin radiation.

April 24, 1985

Well, here we go again. This is day one of radiation. I've got my head together. I'm ready for this new ordeal.

April 25, 1985

The entire radiation session took only about 15 minutes. But it's eerie. I was alone in the radiation room, in my mold on the table. I could see the red light and the machine open like a powerful telescope. Suddenly the buzzer goes off. It screams for an eternity, but it's actually only a few seconds. I simply lie still and let the machine heal me. But it burns the flesh and causes a distinct smell.

This is day two of the new treatment. My arm is already beginning to stiffen. It hurts. But it does seem to feel better after I exercise it a little. I must remember that radiation—like chemotherapy—is really my friend.

April 29, 1985

Al called. We need to talk about financial matters. I know there will be more trouble. And I'll probably need to go to court again. My two battles—with cancer and with my ex-husband—seem endless.

This is day three; only 27 more to go. I still walk when I can. I can love and laugh. But everything in my life right now is iffy. I'm not making any long-range plans.

April 30, 1985

I hate the sound of the buzzer. I hear it in the middle of the night. But spring is here. The warm, lovely days make me want to fight even harder to live. Although this was only day four of radiation, I found it very difficult to walk into that room today. When I was in position on the table, I could only say, "Heal me, baby, heal me."

Thank heavens I have an interior designing job to keep me busy. I'm redoing a dentist's office I first did eight years ago. It will be fun. He's a nice man.

May 1, 1985

I'm one-sixth of the way done. My arm hurts. And I'm very tired. Some people say I have a special glow, but I don't *really* glow in the dark.

There are a lot of nifty people in this department, especially Dr. Per Langeland, my radiologist. All of them encourage their patients.

I would like my whole life to be different, to be calm. I would like to have a little home, a devoted husband, and no excitement. I've had enough excitement for the rest of my life. I say I'd like to try living that way. But I sincerely doubt I could do it for more than two days.

May 2, 1985

I felt sick today as I was driving to the hospital. I parked the car at the far end of the parking lot so I could walk some before I went in for my treatment. It helped.

Some day this will all be behind me. I must be patient and take one day at a time.

May 3, 1985

I heard today that Charlie Loprinzi is leaving. He's going to the Mayo Clinic. I'll miss him. He's been very good to me.

I had dinner tonight with a lady I call my guardian angel. She had been a client at Catalyst and we kept in touch over the years. When she heard about my illness, she called. And, unlike some of my friends who couldn't cope with me and my disease, she rallied around. She is always there when I need help. It's fun to visit her home.

May 6, 1985

As I begin another week of radiation I've learned that I will also face another court battle with Al. Hell! I'd much rather be working at a job 60 hours a week. I'm working to make the biggest profit of all on my balance sheet—life! It's a job that takes everything I've got, 24 hours a day, and a job I barely have energy for.

Some days I think radiation is worse than chemo. I'm alone in that room and in my special mold. I'm alone with my markings and the knowledge that I'm being burned. The smell is awful.

I often joke and kid around with the nurses—it's one way to maintain my sanity. Today I told one of them that a man would lose his way on the roadmap on my chest. The squares and lines are multi-colored. No one would know even if there was a breast under all that. But it's helping to heal me.

May 7, 1985

Today I thought about what I would be like without cancer. But it was unproductive. It's a fantasy and I must deal with reality. I need to get on with my life as it is.

May 8, 1985

Mom and I went out to dinner last night with one of my former professors and his wife, Lewellyn and Gretchen Pfankuchen. It was his 81st birthday. He's a special friend. He was my advisor in political science at the university. When I needed financial aid to finish school after my father died, he helped me get an out-of-state scholarship.

It was great seeing him again. He was happy to be with me. He reminded me that I have a good head on my shoulders and of how well I had done during those college years.

May 9, 1985

Today I had another radiation treatment. I can't get over that feeling of isolation and loneliness that comes over me when I'm left alone in that room. I face the fact that death might be calling. If it does, I'll hang up.

May 10, 1985

There are a few times in everyone's life when it's necessary to stand up to difficult people or situations. I've done it several times. Now the boys have stood up to their father. Next month he's marrying the writer of the love letters I found in April 1980. They told him they will not attend his wedding unless he calls off our court date and signs an agreement to continue paying extra money for my medical needs. I'm sorry the boys have to go through this, but I guess it's part of growing up and living in the adult world.

Their ultimatum worked. The court date is cancelled, and Al has agreed to continue the payments. I'm fighting for my life, and the boys are helping me do that. I want them to learn that it's kindness to people that's important.

May 13, 1985

Yesterday was Mother's Day. I had a fine time with Mom and the boys. Marc and Joel gave me tapes of some of their favorite music, tapes I can play while I'm in radiation and that will remind me that they are with me in spirit. They told me the details of their confrontation with their father. I don't think he has any real notion of what his proposed court action did to his relationship with his sons.

May 15, 1985

I don't know how it's possible, but there seems to be a *third* lump in the same place.

May 18, 1985

It's no surprise, but it's a nuisance. Radiation is messing up my sex life. The area of radiation is very sore. I've been frank about this with the gentleman I'm seeing. He's been great. He's willing to stay with me and adjust to my needs. He's been understanding and patient. He asked, "How many men have the choice of going out with a flat-chested woman or a full-breasted woman?" He answered his own question with, "I have the choice by just turning my head from side to side." I came unglued. Sex is not exactly like it was, but I won't give up the sexual part of my identity. It's part of my life, just as the surgery, drugs, and radiation are. I think sex is a fine medicine too.

May 22, 1985

Today is Joel's 21st birthday, and I had my 18th treatment. I feel lousy. Funny, I'm not usually a willing housekeeper. But cleaning the house has become routine when I feel so rotten. I can work only a few minutes at a time, then I must rest.

The doctors and I discussed the new lump today. They let me make the final decision about surgery. They were pleased when I told them "no surgery." They seem to think it will disappear when I finish radiation.

May 23, 1985

The exhaustion I feel all the time hasn't done a thing to improve my disposition. But I told myself again today that it's okay to break down, to be in a bad mood, to be angry.

As lousy as I felt when I went into that room today, I felt that God was with me. That and the faith that I *will* heal and feel better get me through each session. The machine, God, and me—we're working together for my life.

May 27, 1985

I had a short reprieve from radiation treatments at the end of last week. I went to Minneapolis and met George Bush and his wife, Judy. We went up to see the Metropolitan Opera on tour at Northrop Auditorium on the University of Minnesota campus. We saw *La Boheme*. What a treat!

May 30, 1985

My mood swings are still unpredictable. I detest that room where I have radiation. It has no windows. I can't be in a closed room now. As I spoke to God today I thought about heaven and hell. I firmly believe I will go to heaven because I've spent my time in hell for the past year and a half. But I'm not quite ready even for heaven yet. I need a few more good times and a bit more lovemaking.

May 31, 1985

Yesterday I had my first haircut since December 1983. A haircut! My dear designer cut it quite stylishly. I'm beginning to look like someone I used to know.

June 3, 1985

The end is in sight. This is day 25. I'm hanging on. But dealing with radiation and the exhaustion and depression that come with it is the hardest thing I've ever done. It's difficult even to concentrate on details of the malpractice suit when I meet with Bill.

Later the same day

I've had 25 radiation sessions. I assumed this was routine, until one of the doctors congratulated me. He told me what a success I was: I hadn't quit. But quitting was *never* one of my options. Even on the worst days I knew I had to go through with it. He said I'd done a great job. I told him I want to get on with my life. I'm tired of being sick.

June 5, 1985

I go in for treatment 27 today. I'm burned and bruised. It's hard to move, the pain is so great. It's many times worse than the worst sunburn. The lump seems to have gone down a little.

June 6, 1985

I'm anxious to finish these treatments. My breathing has changed. I was told this might happen but that it would be only temporary. And I can't get rid of that horrible smell.

There is the possibility that I might need more chemotherapy after radiation. I cannot even think rationally about that now. I get tired at the very thought. My skin is very sore. But I am alive.

June 11, 1985

It's almost over. One more day. There were times when I wasn't sure I would make it. But I've managed to keep my mind and body in fairly decent shape.

As much as I want radiation to end, I am scared and confused about finishing. Once again I'll lose a security blanket. But I know I'll be okay.

June 12, 1985

I'm done! Finished! I can hardly believe it. Treatment number 30 was today. How do I feel? Terrific! I made it. I'm alive. They gave me a special certificate in recognition of my great feat. It's neat!

I know I bitched a lot about radiation, the buzzer, the room, everything. But there was one nice thing: a mural showing a field of daisies on one wall of the department waiting room. So, to celebrate the end of my treatments, I sent 30 dozen—360—daisies to the department. I included a note with a special poem about picking daisies. It was written by an

85-year-old woman. The line I like most is "If I had my life to live all over again, I would pick more daisies."

One of the radiologists, Dr. Edward Naill, asked me, "What are you going to do now that this is all wrapped up?" I said, "Just live." Living is my happiness. I just hope for tomorrow and feel lucky to have today.

June 14, 1985

Now that I've had a couple of days to simply *be*, without seeing a doctor or having a treatment of some kind, I'm proud of myself. I've made it through some of the toughest medical procedures known and I'm aching to get on with this business of life.

I have to trust that the chemotherapy and radiation did their jobs. I trust the oncologists, radiologists, and the rest of the medical staff. I know I put my trust in Bob Jackson once, and he betrayed that trust. Nevertheless, I'm unwilling to give up that basic part of me: trust.

And I still have my Purple Tree. It has new branches. The tree is strong. It shades my life and makes me feel secure. The branches bend but they will not break, even when stressed.

June 17, 1985

I was supposed to give my deposition for the malpractice suit at Bill's office today. It was postponed for a month.

I received a wonderful note from all of the nurses who cared for me during radiation. They distributed the flowers around the department.

June 18, 1985

Marc and I took Joel to O'Hare today. He flew to Europe, where he'll spend the summer. I had the disquieting thought that I might not see him again. I must stop thinking like that.

June 24, 1985

I flew to New York yesterday for an appointment with Dr. Cody today. He told me he does not think the newest lump is a tumor. He believes it's scar tissue from surgery and radiation. His advice was to do nothing. He said I am so sore, bruised, and burned from the radiation that there is no way anything can be done for many months.

Now I need time to heal as a woman and as a person. I'll never be free of knowing I have cancer. I hope I won't need further treatment. I'll always fear this insidious disease.

Despite the pain, depression, exhaustion, and other side effects, I would take the same treatments again if it meant the difference between life and death.

CHAPTER 5

June 26, 1985

I've survived cancer thus far. I've survived the chemotherapy. I've survived the recurrence. I've survived 30 radiation treatments. Next I must survive the lawsuit. That's my job now. Fortunately I have the time to concentrate on the case.

I've rekindled my love for jazz. I even joined the Madison Jazz Society. When I listen to jazz I feel more alive.

June 29, 1985

I met with Bill this afternoon to start on one of the most important parts of the lawsuit—my deposition. He explained that a deposition is a transcription of the testimony of a witness adverse to the party taking the deposition. Bob Jackson's attorney will take my deposition. Bill will be there, but he won't ask questions. Similarly, Bill will depose several of Bob's witnesses. Depositions are extremely important because opposing attorneys want to know—before they go to trial—what witnesses on the other side are going to say. They don't like surprises. According to Bill, lawyers usually depose every important witness on the other side in a trial. It is possible to use only the deposition at a trial if for some reason the witness cannot be present.

I'm scared of the lawsuit, but the truth must be told. Bill emphasized that I must not give any more information than is asked for. A good rule is: A thin deposition is a good deposition. The deposition is extremely important because it's a rehearsal of sorts for the hearing. The mere thought of going through all this with only a two percent chance for victory is frightening. Any slight technicality or error in the presentation of a case can change the outcome, no matter how good the case. It doesn't seem to be the ideal way to regain my health. But I must do what is right, and this *is* right.

I find it very difficult not being able to speak to anyone about the lawsuit. I am not known as a woman of few words. In addition, this is an expensive proposition. I'll have to borrow a great deal of money to see this through. The fact that I could go broke will not stop me.

I'm convinced that Bill will do his job well. I don't want him to have to say that if I had just spent a little more I would have won. I couldn't live with that.

July 4, 1985

I had breakfast with Marc in Milwaukee, where he works. We watched "Live Aid" from London knowing Joel was in the crowd. I went to hear a friend play jazz and then took the bus back to Madison.

July 5, 1985

The pressure of preparing to give my deposition is mounting. I'm most apprehensive about two aspects. First, I wonder if I'll be able to handle a long period of discussing my horror; second, I wonder if I'll be able to handle being asked questions I feel are not pertinent.

I met with Bill again this week a couple of times. I taped one of the meetings so I could practice and review the new terminology and my recollections at home. I must be on top of all this. It's part of my survival!

July 17, 1985

Two attorneys for the opposition took my deposition today. Steve Caulum—Bob Jackson's lawyer—could not be there. The attorneys started slowly and worked up to more precise questions.

I got upset only once during the proceedings: when I talked about New York and Dr. Cody's concern for my life and Bob's unbelievably arrogant reaction when I called him that afternoon with my horrifying news. I asked to take a break so I could regain my composure. They asked many questions about my divorce. I gave short answers. We finished about one o'clock.

Bill told me he was proud of my performance. I did well. But I'm tremendously relieved that the deposition is over. Now onward to the real thing!

July 19, 1985

Bill and I have had many discussions about possible witnesses to call for the hearing. We decided to contact my old friend Irving and ask him to testify. I last saw him after my surgery in 1983. Bill called him at his office. He was reluctant to talk to Bill. But he finally did describe to Bill exactly what he'd felt in my breast in 1982 and 1983. However, he refused to testify. He said he doesn't want to get involved. Bill couldn't persuade him to change his mind.

July 20, 1985

It's been a month since I finished my radiation treatments, but my skin still looks scorched. It still hurts too. And—real or imagined—I can still detect that odor of burning flesh.

July 25, 1985

Bill called today to let me know that he's got a good lead to someone who might be our expert witness for the hearing. He expects to make contact with this doctor soon.

August 5, 1985

Marc will be moving to St. Louis later this month. He has a new job with an ad agency. I'll miss his being so close. But I know I'll enjoy visiting him in St. Louis. He likes the idea of being back in Missouri, where he went to college.

Next it will be Joel. Then, if I live, I'll move. But first things first. I need to finish the lawsuit and I need to be with Dr. Carbone and his treatments for cancer—his "basket of goodies," as he calls them.

It's tough to realize that I can't make long-term plans. No one can. I just learned it faster than most.

August 10, 1985

I'm not getting along with Bill. It seems we're always at odds these days. He's going through a rough divorce. And at times he's preoccupied with his personal life. It's difficult for him, but this lawsuit is all-important to me. I feel for him about the divorce. I've been there. But he must decide about my case. I'm thinking of seeing someone else, even though I don't want to hire another attorney. The delay could be harmful, and the cost prohibitive.

August 16, 1985

I told Bill that I'm meeting with another Madison lawyer today to review my case. I definitely do not want to change lawyers again. But if Bill doesn't begin to pay more attention to my case, this new man could take over. He too thinks I have a strong case. If I've learned anything from my experience with cancer, it's to get a second opinion. I also talked with Clifford and Relles. They advised me not to change, that my having these doubts is natural. They know I'm not feeling well, that maybe Bill and I just need time to work this out. I'll meet with Bill again in a couple of weeks.

August 21, 1985

Bill met with the lawyer I had contacted on August 16. Bill talked about the case as he sees it and about what he has done so far. Very shortly I'll be at the point of no return: I must make up my mind about which attorney will represent me. I want help but, as with my cancer, I'm the only one who can make this decision. The second attorney said he would work with Bill if I wanted him to or he could take over. However, he says Bill is doing a fine job. Once I make this decision, I will stick with it and not try to second-guess Bill.

August 24, 1985

I'm picking Joel up in Chicago today. He's been in Europe all summer. Marc will meet us at the O'Hare Hyatt. The three of us will be together again. I feel very safe when the boys are with me. God, I love them.

August 26, 1985

Joel looks tired and a bit thin but very grown up. The boys and I discussed some of the problems with the lawsuit. They think I should stay with Bill. But they urged me to tell him my feelings about the case and his handling of it. They think—and I know they're right—that Bill and I must be completely honest with each other if we are to get on with it and win this case.

August 28, 1985

Bill talked with Dr. Harvey Golomb yesterday. He's the potential expert witness Bill told me about last month. Dr. Golomb is an oncologist/hematologist at the University of Chicago Hospital and Medical School. Bill wrote him about my case and asked if he'd be willing to testify. Dr. Golomb called Bill and said he was interested, but needed my medical records. Bill has sent everything to the doctor.

September 3, 1985

Hurray! Dr. Golomb will be my expert witness. He called Bill at home over the weekend and agreed.

September 9, 1985

When I got to Bill's office today, he told me I must choose now. Will it be him or someone else representing me? I wasn't quite ready to give him an answer. But I do know there will be only one lawyer representing me when the hearing begins. I promised him that I'll decide very soon.

September 10, 1985

I met with my banker, David Mergen, today. I need financial help to see this lawsuit through to its conclusion. He was most helpful. I put up my house for collateral. I told him I would do whatever was necessary to obtain a line of credit to finance the suit. He was most understanding. There was no hassle.

There's no turning back now. If I lose, I'll move into an apartment.

September 24, 1985

Bill and I had a long talk today. I think he finally understands me. I hope I understand him. He knows I want justice. He wants to win. He'll focus on my case for the next few months. Suddenly we're a team again. It's essential for me to know that he's committed to me and my case.

As I look back at this episode, I think it was not all bad. It helped us cement the client/attorney relationship. We needed to reaffirm our allegiance to each other to be a winning team.

September 25, 1985

Bill called. He had prepared a letter to send to Bob's attorney, Steve Caulum, offering to settle the case out of court. We had discussed this and Bill knew that I was worried about the cost of pursuing the case, both in terms of money and in terms of my health.

October 11, 1985

Bill and Bob's attorney, Steve Caulum, went to Chicago yesterday to depose Dr. Harvey Golomb, my expert witness.

Bill sounded very pleased when he called today. He is certain Dr. Golomb will be a convincing witness for me. He told me he was still somewhat overwhelmed by what happened when he and Steve met with Dr. Golomb.

As Bill tells it, when they arrived at the doctor's office, Dr. Golomb came "flying in." His nurse told him the two attorneys from Madison were there to see him, by appointment. Dr. Golomb said something like, "Oh, yes, I have to talk with you today. Come in."

Bill went into the office with the doctor for what was supposed to be a private five-minute talk before the deposition started. In that brief period, Bill says, the doctor took and made several phone calls, dealing with both business and private matters. He also conferred with his nurse about a couple of patient calls. When Bill finally got his undivided attention, it was just about time for Steve to come in and begin taking his deposition.

At that point, Bill says, he was amazed to see a remarkable transformation take place. Dr. Golomb visibly slowed down, sat up straight in his chair, and said he was ready. When Bill protested that he needed a few minutes to brief him, the doctor said, "Just be cool. I know what I'm doing. I've done this before. Just be cool. All right?" Bill did as he was told. He had no choice.

And, to quote Bill further, "The doctor was cool. He was one of the most articulate men I have ever heard as he reviewed the material and answered Steve's questions. He was totally organized. He was terrific. I felt better and better as we went along."

Bill's excitement is contagious. After that conversation I feel a lot more confident about my case.

November 4, 1985

Marc is 25 years old today. It's hard to believe. I'm flying down to St. Louis to celebrate in a few days. He wants me there as his mom and his interior designer. I'm helping him with his new apartment.

November 6, 1985

I was interviewed today by Les Goldsmith, a vocational expert. He will testify at the hearing. He questioned me about my working life and my abilities. He will calculate what my earnings could have been. He's very nice, a sensitive and competent man. After the interview, I realized how much I loved being in business and how much I miss it.

November 14, 1985

I had my regular bi-monthly appointment with Dr. Carbone this morning. Hurray! No new lumps, even though I do have a case of shingles. Dr. Carbone assured me it's probably a result of my exhaustion from chemotherapy and radiation and the tension and stress connected with the lawsuit. He wished me luck. I appreciate his support.

November 15, 1985

Today I saw Fred Coleman. He and Wil Fey will testify next week in the hearing. Nice people. I can't imagine what I would have done without their help and excellent therapy. It all goes together—the medicine, the body, and the head.

As I reviewed the list of people who have helped so far and those who will help by testifying at the hearing, I decided to try once more to persuade Irving to appear as a witness. In a letter dated July 30, 1985, he advised me to forget about the lawsuit, to "talk to your doctor and settle it with a handshake." But at this point—four days before the hearing was to start—Bill and I hoped he might change his mind, especially if he knew more of the facts about my case. So I called his office. I learned he was out of town on business. After half a dozen calls I tracked him down in Bismarck, North Dakota. I asked him to reconsider his decision. I appealed to him on the ground that he knew the truth and could help me. He wouldn't budge. He will not be a witness.

November 16, 1985

Today it was my radiologist's turn. I'm okay. My skin feels better, but I'm still exhausted. Will I ever not be?

November 18, 1985

The hearing begins tomorrow. My case will be heard by a Patient Compensation Panel. The State Supreme Court controls the panels through the office of the Director of Courts, as provided in a 1975 state law. Each five-member panel consists of two physicians (or one physician and one other health care provider), two public members, and one attorney who serves as chair. The Director of Courts selects the medical people from lists submitted by "appropriate statewide organizations" and public members from a list submitted by the governor.

Each side can request the removal of one panel member. And each side can strike one attorney's name from the list of three submitted by the Director of Courts. The Director also chooses the hearing site.

The panel must decide, according to the statute: 1) Whether the actions or omissions of the health care provider were negligent; and 2) If such actions or omissions were negligent, whether that negligence caused injury or death to the patient.

After the panel announces its decision, both sides have 60 days to appeal for a circuit court trial.

I'm scared. So is Bill. But he assures me he's well prepared. I believe him. He also told me that Steve Caulum had never answered his letter in which we offered to settle the case. Dave Relles called to wish us luck. He was reassuring and said we have a great case. He's sure both Bill and I are ready. I've gone over and over the specific dates and procedures, the whole truth. It will be in my head forever.

It was my lump, my cancer, my breast. It's my body, my life.

CHAPTER 6 *

November 19, 1985

Marc called early this morning to give me a pep talk and to wish me well. Joel drove me to the Ramada Inn on the east side where the hearing is being held. I was there well before the 8 A.M. starting time. Joel had classes this morning, so he couldn't stay long. Once again I was alone, facing the unknown. And once again I was scared.

But there was a difference. I went into this five-day ordeal with a sense of inner peace. I knew I was doing the right thing. But, unlike my ordeal with cancer, *I* was in control of the decision to sue. In addition, I knew Bill was well prepared. He had left nothing to chance. And he had prepared me for my part in the hearing. I knew that I had to be strong. I knew that when it was my turn to testify I had to tell—as Jack Webb from "Dragnet" used to say—"just the facts."

I believed we had a winning case. But there were moments when I wondered if justice would be done. I wondered if my testimony would contribute to the success or the failure of the hearing. And I wondered if Bill would achieve his hopes or fall short. I'll know the answers by the end of this week.

I don't know what I had expected when I walked into the hearing room. Maybe I thought there would be more of a

*Quotations in this chapter from Diane Craig Chechik's hearing before the Patient Compensation Panel are taken from official transcripts. Grammar, punctuation, and capitalization reflect that of the transcripts.

Perry Mason atmosphere. I was sure these proceedings would be more dramatic than the divorce-related matters for which I had been to court previously.

Room 299 is a typical motel conference room. I have no idea why this particular place was chosen for the hearing. Perhaps it's convenient for all involved. As I surveyed the room for the first time, I mentally began to redecorate. Carpet, wallpaper, draperies, and furniture are in varying and unmatched designs and in shades of green and rust.

At one end of the rectangular room three long tables were set up in the shape of a U. The center table was where the panel would sit. To their right was the defense table, facing the windows that overlook the parking lot and East Washington Avenue. To the left was our table; I would be facing Bob Jackson throughout the hearing. In between these two tables was the witness chair. A projector, easel for exhibits, and blackboard were also in the room for use during the hearing. To my right was the place for the court reporter. A pitcher of water, glasses, and a piece of peppermint candy for each person were on each table. In the back of the room there were chairs for witnesses waiting to testify and for the public. Coffee was also available on a table in the back of the room.

All in all, the mood of the room was somber and serious. It not only fit the gray of the weather outdoors, it was a good match for the seriousness of the business at hand. I wore a plain gray four-piece outfit—skirt, shirt, vest, and jacket, perfect for the occasion. I wore only one piece of jewelry, the family ring.

Bob was there, looking very professional and wearing his perennial bow tie. Then I got my first look at defense attorney Steve Caulum. He's quite tall, probably six foot three or four, good-looking, and has a full head of dark hair. He looked very confident. Both he and Bill were conservatively dressed in dark suits. Bill is not much over five foot eight and is balding.

The panel for my hearing is chaired by Leo Hansen, a Beloit attorney. Others on the panel are Drs. Ralph Kennedy of Appleton and Thomas Ries of Sheboygan; and public members Gwen Gunderson of Portage and Marvin Kaukl of Poynette.

Chairman Hansen instructed attorneys and witnesses on the procedures to be followed. We were ready to begin. I looked across the room at Bob. Our eyes met. We looked at each other for a moment. We both wondered what the outcome would be, and I wondered if justice would be done.

The first witness to testify was Bob Jackson. Bill called him as an adverse witness. Bill had explained his strategy as "wanting to make sure there wasn't going to be any question about your reliability, Diane, in showing up as a patient. I wanted to try to rebut any contributory negligence claim. They were going to say you were supposed to come in regularly. I needed specific information about the regularity of your visits. I needed his descriptions of your visits."

Bill got that information as he took Bob back over my records from the time I became his patient in 1968. His records showed I had been in for an examination—including a breast exam—almost every year. Apparently in the early seventies I skipped a year twice. Otherwise I was in to see him very regularly, and my breast exams were normal, according to his records.

In the course of his testimony Bob described as "indistinct" or "unclear" what he felt when he examined me. He said those descriptions are "different than cancer" and that cancer is very distinct. Bill knew, however, from the literature plus a couple of depositions that many experts disagree with that statement. They all said that cancer can be indistinct. Bill told me that he felt very good about the results of his medical research. The people who wrote the books and treatises, he said, "had no reason to be biased. They don't know us. But they come out on our side." Bill wanted Bob's answers on the record so they couldn't be changed when Bill introduced his information from the literature.

Bill also got Bob to admit that cancer was a "possibility" when he examined me in March 1982. Further, Bob admitted that in November 1983 he knew that cancer was "high on one's list."

Bill will have another chance to question Bob Jackson later, in cross examination.

I was the next witness. Although Bill thought I was well prepared and ready to testify, he wasn't taking any chances. He wanted me on and off the stand, as he put it, "because I wanted to be able to gauge and repair any damage you might do." He knew I was under a great deal of tension. Just sitting in that hearing room was stressful. And, having heard only one witness so far talk about me, I was beginning to find it very distasteful. Testifying was without doubt one of the most nerve-wracking and exhausting experiences I've had.

My testimony began with a description of what the lump felt like and what was said and done during each visit to Bob Jackson. The hardest part of my testimony occurred when Bill entered into evidence pictures of me, first the one taken in 1982 and then one from 1984 when I was completely bald. I nearly cried. I had to hold the pictures as I talked about them.

At that point, Steve requested permission to ask me a question. Panel chair Leo Hansen granted it.

"Did you have these pictures taken for the hearing?" Steve asked.

I closed my eyes and swallowed hard. I had to keep my cool. I looked at him incredulously and said, "No!" Panel members were examining copies of these same pictures. They seemed to look at Steve as if to ask, "How could you do that to this woman?"

Later Bill described how I reacted to the situation. "It was very real. You just looked back on who you were and I could see, by what you were experiencing, that you felt some really deep hurt about what had happened here. This was a bold, graphic description of where you were then and where you are now."

Bill told me at the end of this incredible day, "You were terrific. You were believable, you were honest. And I don't think you angered them at any point. You were flawless."

Bill's praise was exactly what I needed after several hours on the witness stand. I understand now why many people—even victims of crimes—are reluctant to get involved in court cases. It's an experience I wouldn't wish on anyone.

As I write this tonight, I realize that throughout the day, and especially when I was on the witness stand, I held on for dear life to the braided rope belt on my skirt. Somehow I knew that if I could keep my hands still, I'd be under control. In the other hand I clutched a linen hankie. I wanted to be ready if the tears came.

November 20, 1985

My psychologist, Wil Fey, was the first witness this morning. This wonderful man, whom I began consulting when I was getting my divorce, is soft-spoken and very gentle. Bill wanted him to testify about the psychological effect on me of the delay in diagnosing cancer. Wil told the panel that my anger was intensified by the fact that I knew it didn't have to be this way.

Bill had told me that would be the argument for "pain and suffering. Not only have you endured the pain and suffering, you've had to live with the knowledge that you needn't have endured that pain and suffering."

Wil also testified that I was angry about my situation very early on—before the lawsuit. My anger was not the invention of a lawyer who wanted to make money on my malpractice suit. He emphasized that my anger was an immediate reaction when I learned my doctor had missed the malignancy.

Panel member Dr. Thomas Ries asked Wil what kind of notes he kept on our consultations. Wil told him he doesn't keep notes; everything is in his head. Dr. Ries asked how he could do things that way. Wil came back with, "You practice your way, and I'll practice my way."

Vocational expert Les Goldsmith was called as our next witness. He simply testified about my potential earning capacity.

My next three witnesses did not testify in person. Drs. Paul Carbone and John Pellett gave their testimony via video tape; Dr. Hiram Cody's testimony was taken on the telephone and taped. Both sides had agreed to use these electronic vehicles for presenting their testimony. However, none could testify as to Bob's negligence or liability; they were not named as expert witnesses.

Even before the hearing began, Bill was pleased with the statements my three doctors had made. Dr. Carbone went first. He testified about the treatments I had received at the University of Wisconsin Clinical Cancer Center. He described and explained details of chemotherapy and radiation. Members of the panel were familiar with his international reputation in oncology. This gentle, caring, grandfatherly man is not only my doctor; he has become a good friend. I couldn't help thinking as he testified that Dr. Carbone's other great passion is bicycling. If he can't bike 80 to 100 miles at a time, it's not a real trip. He always tells me—everyone, in fact—that when he finds a cure for cancer, he's going to retire from medicine and open a bicycle repair shop. This wonderful man's brain is keeping me alive.

Bill was most impressed by Dr. Carbone. "What I liked most about him was his manner. He is very likable and believable. I think he won over the panel. That was really beneficial."

Dr. John Pellett, the next witness, is a skilled surgeon who is genuinely concerned about his patients' welfare. Bill felt that Dr. Pellett "showed that his way of treating a possible malignancy in the breast was different from Jackson's." I thought once again about how lucky I was to have a doctor of that caliber for my surgeon.

Dr. Cody, who was heard on tape, would have made quite an impression on the panel if he'd been there in person. He is about six foot four, slender, with a beautiful smile and thinning light-colored hair. He exudes an aura of professionalism. His voice was authoritative as he said that the cancer was clearly there in November. Bill and I both felt that he came off well.

.   .   .

I met our expert witness, Dr. Harvey Golomb, for the first time this afternoon. He's a handsome, medium-sized man in his 40s. He was very dapper in a gray ultrasuede jacket and suede shoes.

Dr. Golomb was just simply terrific. First of all, his credentials are first-rate. He is Director of the Joint Section on Hematology/Oncology, University of Chicago Medical Center and Michael Reese Medical Center. He is also a full professor of medicine at the University of Chicago. He has written and published 216 articles and texts. And he has testified for both plaintiffs and defendants in medical malpractice suits. Bill was especially pleased with that because the experts on the other side had all testified only for defendants. As he put it, "Here was someone who will take either side and state his opinion. I *was* a little worried about his patient-care responsibility. But I found out when we took the deposition that he actually does see a fairly large number of patients."

Bill took Dr. Golomb quickly through testimony about his having reviewed all the medical records related to my case. On direct examination by Bill, Dr. Golomb discussed Bob's record of March 29, 1982, the day he did the needle aspiration. (Bill had some of Bob's records blown up for use at the hearing. They were put on the easels during several parts of the proceedings and were visible to everyone in the room.)

Dr. Golomb's testimony was quite technical. I've included the parts I consider vital to my case. He was our expert witness.

Q. Doctor, did you review the record of March 29, 1982?

A. Yes, sir.

Q. And based upon those records did it appear to you that Dr. Jackson examined . . . or saw Mrs. Chechik on that day?

A. Yes, sir.

Q. And what were his findings on that day?

A. . . . I went through the findings. They're based on the drawing . . . as well as the procedure that he did, which was needle aspiration, which he noted to be negative.

He did order a mammogram, and he also noted an impression of mammary hyperplasia.

Q. Now the notation negative needle aspiration, what did you understand that to mean?

A. I understood that to mean . . . that something in this area was felt to be abnormal and that a needle was stuck into that and that nothing was obtained. No fluid was obtained.

Q. And, Doctor, . . . impression, mammary hyperplasia, what did you understand that to mean?

A. I understood that was Dr. Jackson's impression of what this abnormality was in the breast . . . although mammary hyperplasia by definition is a pathologic term, not a clinical term.

Q. Could you explain to the panel what that means when you say it is a pathologic term?

A. Well, a pathologic term is . . . a description of something seen under the microscope whereas a clinical term is something that we would feel or see.

So we might say since we didn't have a microscope here . . . to look at this, . . . an impression might have said breast irregularity, or breast firmness, or irregular mass, . . . but mammary hyperplasia as such is really a pathological diagnosis.

Q. Is it possible to make that diagnosis, mammary hyperplasia, based upon palpation?

A. No.

Dr. Golomb confirmed that he had read Dr. Davis's March 30, 1982, mammogram report. Bill asked the witness for his interpretation.

A. Well, the essence of that mammogram report was that there was an increased density in the upper outer quadrants of both breasts where the appearance [of] a lesion could be obscured. . . .

And then a subsequent statement was made clinically if a mass is felt on the right it should be biopsied, suggesting to me that the mammographer was suspicious of something but wanted to correlate that . . . with the clinical findings. . . .

In this case what would have been indicated would have been an excisional biopsy of this area. Not only would it have been indicated from the mammogram report, but the fact that the negative needle aspiration was obtained is also more support for doing an excisional biopsy. So we have two things at that point that should have moved Dr. Jackson to consider an excisional biopsy of the patient at that time.

Dr. Golomb told the panel that a needle aspiration is called for if there is a "palpable irregularity in the breast." If no fluid is obtained from the lesion, "then the chance of it being a solid tumor are much higher." He went on to explain that a "solid" tumor does not necessarily mean a malignant tumor. But, he added, "you can't differentiate by the feel . . .whether this is a benign or malignant tumor. . . ."

Bill then turned to my second visit to Bob's office on June 29, 1982. He asked the witness if, in his opinion, "to a reasonable degree of medical certainty," Dr. Jackson "exercised the . . . degree of care, skill, and judgment which is usually exercised under like or similar circumstances," and if the advanced state of medical science at that time had been taken into account.

A. I think the fact that he identified the finding in the breast to be the same as before and referred to it as a mass tells me . . . that, regardless of what the mammogram showed at that time, . . . there was still an abnormality which was persistent over a three-month period of time.

We all know that there is a 15 to 20 percent false negative rate in mammograms, and that this patient should have gone on to have an excisional biopsy at that time.

So, not only was it missed, the procedure should have been done in March and April. But the second chance was also lost in June or July of '82.

In response to Bill's question about what a breast cancer feels like, Dr. Golomb said "there can be a range of feelings of breast cancer" and added:

A. Frequently the smaller abnormalities are somewhat indistinct and it's almost a suspicion that it's different from the rest of the breast, and that you have to have a high index of suspicion that you could be dealing with something malignant.

At this point, only part way through Dr. Golomb's testimony, I was feeling good about my case. Then Bill came in with what I have labeled a series of "blockbuster" questions.

He asked Dr. Golomb if he had an opinion as to "whether or not cancer was present in Diane Chechik's right breast in March of 1982."

A. My opinion is that it was most probably present in the breast in March of '82. And that is based on the fact that there was an abnormality noted in this drawing in March of '82. That the same abnormality was confirmed in June of '82, and subsequently when Dr. Cody examined the patient in November of '82 [sic] as well as Dr. Jackson just prior to Dr. Cody and subsequently, before he referred the patient to University of Wisconsin Hospital, that the location of an abnormality was always in the exact same quadrant of the breast, this right upper outer quadrant of the breast.

So . . . with the persistence of this finding in March and June, and the subsequent examinations, my opinion is that this was the same abnormality and that it was breast cancer back in early '82.

The next couple of questions elicited the information that a breast lesion is "usually" palpable when it's about one centimeter in size.

Q. And according to the medical record what was the size of this malignancy at the time it was removed?

A. Oh, at the time of removal there were two things. One is the clinical measurements which were what we referred to in terms of palpating it, and Dr. Cody noted that the mass in the upper outer quadrant was 3 by 3.5 centimeters, and the University of Wisconsin examiner on 12/15/83 noted that it was 4 by 4 centimeters. . . . 4 by 4 centimeters is almost like a good-sized golf ball.

Dr. Golomb went on to explain that the area of the breast where cancer most frequently occurs is the upper outer quadrant, exactly where mine was.

Bill came right back with more blockbuster questions.

Q. Doctor, in order to be within the standard of care that is . . . usually exercised by a like or similar physician, is it necessary to eliminate cancer as a possibility when faced with a dominant mass, if we call it that?

A. I think if one felt that there was an abnormality that was not symmetrical from one breast to the . . . other, and certainly when the breast was atypical in one quadrant compared to the others, that the possibility of this being cancer is extremely high.

It's the only major lethal disease of the breast and must be considered in the work-up and carried to completion, which usually includes excisional biopsy.

Seven out of eight excisional biopsies are frequently not cancer but they're worth doing for the one out of eight which turn out to be cancer.

Q. . . . Is it necessary . . . to be within the standard of care for a physician to eliminate cancer as a possibility when faced with a breast abnormality?. . .

A. Yes, sir.

Q. And does it matter whether that abnormality is labeled a dominant mass or not a dominant mass?

A. I think the question of dominant mass is semantics in a way. If there is an abnormality that is asymmetrical then it's one we have to be concerned about.

Q. Doctor, in order to be within that standard of care, would it be acceptable for . . . a 5 percent chance of cancer being present?

A. I certainly would not be content with explaining . . . to a patient that there was a 5 percent chance. I think for that 5 percent I would want to do the excisional biopsy. . . .

Q. Doctor, the question is in order for a physician to be within the standard of care when faced with a breast abnormality in March of 1982 is it acceptable to have a 5 percent chance of cancer?

A. No.

Q. What is acceptable?

A. I think no chance with a breast that's easy to biopsy.

Dr. Golomb said that he is not a mammographer, but he has ordered mammograms as "an aid in trying to decide . . .whether or not I need to biopsy or how soon."

He went on, ". . . if I feel something within the breast, I'm probably going to biopsy it no matter what the mammogram shows."

Bill's next few questions dealt with the reliability of mammograms in diagnosing breast cancer. Dr. Golomb said that various studies report 75 percent to about 85 percent accuracy. He stated that he doesn't think mammography alone should replace biopsy when a physician finds a breast abnormality.

A. . . . the record . . . clearly says the physician felt something abnormal, and even with a negative mammogram the fact that something abnormal was felt, and a needle was stuck in, was enough to move on to the next step which was to do an excisional biopsy to show that cancer was there. At the time it was small hopefully and hadn't spread.

Next, Dr. Golomb quoted from an article in *The Archives of Surgery* by Dr. Donald L. Morton, chief of surgical oncology at UCLA. The article was titled "Delayed Diagnosis of Breast Cancer as a Result of Normal Mammograms."

Steve objected to using the article as evidence because it was published in 1983 and the mammograms in question were made a year earlier.

Leo Hansen overruled the objection, saying that "unless it's shown that the standard of care changed from '82 to '83, it's certainly admissible." Dr. Golomb demolished the objection completely when he pointed out that the article had been "accepted for publication on August 4, 1982. And wasn't published until '83."

He explained that the article did not deal with the reliability of mammograms. Rather it presented data dealing only with the "question of what a delay of using a normal mammogram means to the progression of the disease. . . . they do make a statement for example mammography should not be used to avoid biopsy of a clinically suspicious lesion, which is one of the issues that we have in this case."

His testimony about the article included the fact that the author advocates an excisional biopsy for masses that prove to be non-cystic—that means no fluid—as in my case.

Quoting from the article, Dr. Golomb read, "At no time should a normal mammogram be interpreted to mean that biopsy is not indicated in patients with a clinically suspicious mass."

Then Bill asked another critical question.

Q. Doctor, I believe you have already rendered an opinion that Diane Chechik did have cancer in her breast in March of 1982. I'm asking now . . . whether or not you have an opinion that that cancer was diagnosable?

A. Yes. It was diagnosable since it was noted by the physician in his record.

Q. And again, how would that have been diagnosed?

A. It would have required an excisional biopsy at that time.

Dr. Golomb's testimony was serving to confirm that I was right in bringing this suit against Bob Jackson. Although I knew we still had a long way to go, I felt better and more calm. I felt I had a chance.

Bill suggested that I leave the room for the remainder of Dr. Golomb's testimony. As he said later, "I knew that having you sit here while the witness talked about your chances of surviving would just be too cruel. It would have implied that we'd do anything to win this case.

"After you left the room I told the witness I wanted to talk about the effect of a delay in diagnosis in this particular case.

"Dr. Golomb's answers to a series of questions about the 'staging concept' of breast cancer confirmed that you had a Stage Two tumor with lymph node involvement by the time you had surgery in 1983.

"The witness used charts and the blackboard to illustrate the points he made about staging, lymph node involvement, and relapse rates. He cited a lot of statistical data and concluded, 'By the time she was diagnosed at 12/83 we were almost certain that she was going to end up relapsing by 10 years. She is very unfortunate because she ended up relapsing within a year and a half.'

"According to Dr. Golomb's figures, your condition put you in a category where 65 percent of the patients relapse by five years and 92 percent by 10 years.

"When I heard the answer to my next question, I was awfully glad you weren't in the room.

Q. Doctor, after a relapse what effect does a relapse have on someone's life expectancy?

A. Unfortunately, in breast cancer once the patient relapses they'll never be cured. It's an unalterable course to death.

"He discussed briefly the advances being made in treatment. He said the relapse rate can be cut in half with the sort of chemotherapy you received. He continued:

A. This patient had that kind of therapy and still relapsed . . . six months after she stopped. So she fell into the . . . 33 percent of patients who are still going to relapse even with treatment. And it's unfortunate that she came to this point because if she were possibly diagnosed in 3/82 and had the surgery, there is a very reasonable chance that she would have had no lymph node involvement and would [not] have had this type of prognosis and might not have recurred.

"Then I asked what your life expectancy is now—based upon the cancer you had, the chemotherapy you had, and the relapse in April of 1985.

A. Well, the relapse she had in April of 1985 was a chest wall relapse. And although we frequently want to hope that this is a very local thing . . . we usually understand that this is the tip of the iceberg. . . .

But I think she'll have evidence of systemic relapse probably within the next year or two. I think the major message is to understand once that disease recurs that the patient will never be cured of the disease.

"The doctor went on to quote more statistics about life expectancy. He ended this part of his testimony with these somber words:

A. . . . I don't have a crystal ball, but I did not underemphasize the fact that since she has recurred that she's going to have continual problems with this and eventually die of this disease.

"On that note, I turned the witness over to Steve for cross examination. Dr. Golomb was unshakeable. The defense could not get him to qualify or contradict anything he had said on direct examination. They could not trip him up.

"After questions from members of the panel and some redirect examination by me, he delivered what I guess I would call the knockout punch in response to a question from Leo Hansen:

Q. Is it a proper conclusion . . . if no fluid comes out when you aspirate that there is no abnormality there?

A. No. That's probably the crux of the whole issue here, and that's probably the thing that I've tried to emphasize I'm most critical of . . . the fact that the aspiration was done, no fluid was obtained, and the physician did not advise the patient to go on to have a biopsy at that time.

"Dr. Golomb was indeed a cool customer. He was just simply a sensational witness. The fact that he gave an opinion on negligence was truly of great significance to our case. The best part of his testimony was not all of those charts, but the fact that he stood at the blackboard as a lecturer. All of the people in that room had been in school, and you do tend to believe your teachers. He was the one expert who gave the appearance of being an objective teacher, the professor who was explaining things. He had all eyes on him while he went through this. His manner was what I liked most. He captured their attention and held it. Let's hope the rest of our witnesses do as well."

I returned to the hearing room after Dr. Golomb had left the witness stand. Bill told me his impression of our expert witness, and I was relieved, to say the least, that things had worked out so well.

Our last witness of the day was my psychiatrist, Fred Coleman. He gave straightforward testimony that reinforced Wil's. In addition to painting a second picture of my pain and suffering, he described very graphically the impact that chemotherapy, the recurrence, and the radiation had on me. I think the panel was impressed with the case he made, despite the fact that they may have been taken aback at first by the appearance of this thoroughly professional man who wears a braid down the back of his head. But he knows his business and I don't know what I would do without him.

November 21, 1985

As I drove out to the Ramada Inn this morning, I knew this was going to be a very tough day. Bob

Jackson would be on the witness stand this afternoon. But, in a way, I was looking forward to it. I wanted to hear what kind of a story he'd tell.

Dr. Rudy Hecht was our only witness this morning. He is an older man—reminds me of Santa Claus—and is partly retired. Dr. Hecht was head of family practice at the University of Wisconsin Hospital.

He did three very important things for us. First, he was able to, as Bill said, "put our treatises in evidence. That way it would be the opinions in the treatises for the panel to consider."

At lunch, Bill told me that Dr. Hecht had confirmed that the treatises are authoritative. "I had him enter a lot of articles, so he was able to say that he agreed with them.

"Dr. Hecht explained that an important part of the defense case was that you had a mammogram on two occasions. And all of the information that he introduced from the medical texts established that mammograms are about 90 percent effective—they don't detect one out of 10 tumors. I wanted that figure—one out of 10—underlined, so to speak. It was important because it continues to say that mammograms aren't to be used as the only diagnostic technique because they miss too high a percentage. All of Jackson's experts had to agree with that, and they did.

"Another wonderful thing we got from Dr. Hecht," Bill said, "was the video tape. You weren't here when we showed it. It was a Continuing Medical Education telecourse titled *Malignancy No. 1 in Women—Breast Cancer Management in the 1980s*. It featured Drs. Carbone, Richard Love, and William Wolberg, all on the University of Wisconsin Clinical Cancer Center staff.

"Well," Bill continued, "the beauty of it was one question asking what the doctor should do when faced with a 'negative mammogram and a suspicious lesion?' There were four options: 'a) order repeat mammogram; b) have the patient return for follow-up in six weeks; c) order ultrasound; d) biopsy the lesion.' And right there—in living color—is Dr. Carbone giving the answer, 'biopsy the lesion.' "

Dr. Hecht had one final contribution to make. He had brought with him the instruments used for needle aspirations and needle biopsies. He wanted the panel to understand the difference between the two procedures as well as to show how easy it was to take a needle biopsy.

The instruments were examined by members of the panel as the doctor explained how they are used. In a needle aspiration fluid is taken from the breast, while in a needle biopsy a tissue sample is taken.

I think that actually seeing these instruments helped clarify some of the medical terminology, especially for the non-medical members of the panel. Seeing those two different needles reminded me of why I was here. Bob did not perform a needle biopsy on me. But the procedure is so simple I don't see how it could have failed to impress the panel.

· · ·

Bob was the first witness this afternoon. I had spent most of the noon hour steeling myself to sit through his testimony. I was determined not to lose my composure.

His testimony began with a resume of his professional qualifications and a statement that when I consulted him he was an employee of Madison Obstetrics and Gynecology, Ltd. He said he has been on the University of Wisconsin staff since 1961 as a clinical instructor, assistant clinical professor, and, finally, associate clinical professor. That involves his working with and lecturing to medical students and residents. He pointed out that he has never been paid for this work; his salary comes from his private practice. (Clinical professors are unpaid. The word "clinical" is deleted in describing fulltime, paid staff members at the University of Wisconsin.)

Bob's testimony on direct examination was no surprise. He said exactly what we expected: that he had done nothing wrong, that what he felt in my breast in 1982 was not a malignant tumor.

He did say that in 1982 he thought I might have a 10 percent chance of having cancer. That got to me. Apparently it never occurred to him to let *me* in on that bit of information, to give *me* the option of deciding whether or not to have further tests or a biopsy. I could hear him say again in his strong, professional tone, "Diane, you don't have cancer."

They made much of the fact that I had received a card from his office reminding me to make an appointment. I never received or even saw one of those cards, and I had so testified.

Things got rather confused at this point. Bob had just finished his direct testimony. Then, because Bill's cross examination would take so long, the panel called Dr. Mackman for both his direct and cross examinations. He is a well-known and highly respected surgeon at the Jackson Clinic and Methodist Hospital. Bill will cross examine Bob tomorrow. Bill told me that this slight change in the order of witnesses meant he would have the whole night to prepare for his questioning of Bob Jackson in the morning.

Dr. Mackman's testimony supported Bob's claim that he had done nothing wrong. He said that Bob is an experienced and reputable physician and wasn't negligent.

At this point Leo Hansen said he had some questions for Mackman. At first they appeared to be innocuous. Then they got more and more penetrating.

Q. . . . You mentioned something that I would like to have an answer on, Doctor, if you can. You indicated your decision with regard to an opinion of . . . no negligence by Dr. Jackson was the fact that you know his reputation and you know his experience and that's an important factor to you?

A. That is correct.

Q. So your opinion in this case is based somewhat . . . on the fact that you know the man who did the examining?

A. Yes, I think if you took a rookie right out of medical school . . . it might be a little different situation. . . . It's based on his experience, partly.

Q. Now, if you had a blank on the name of all the records given to you and you didn't know who the examining physician was, would your opinion have been the same? . . .

A. . . . I probably would have just refused to testify in either case because I wouldn't have had enough information.

Bill looked like the proverbial cat who has just swallowed the canary. He leaned over and whispered that he thought Dr. Mackman had as much as said that he would not be here testifying if Bob Jackson wasn't a good friend of his. Then he gave a thumbs-up sign under the table.

But Leo Hansen wasn't through with Dr. Mackman yet. He had a few questions about my visit to Bob on November 21, 1983.

Q. In the report of Dr. Jackson on 11/21/83, he says very clearly two breast masses, one in the beginning of the right axilla and the other in the outer quadrant. Now, does that tell you that there is a probability of cancer?

A. . . . if I just saw that it would make it much more ominous.

Q. And with that and [what] you saw as a clinical examiner, would you wait more than a day or two to re-examine or to take an aspiration or a biopsy or whatever is necessary?

A. I don't think the delay has any real significance.

Q. . . . assuming this was just the first exam that was ever conducted, no mastectomy, you don't know a thing about it . . . would this have alerted you to have a further testing almost immediately?

A. Yes, taken . . . in the abstract, but . . . she was planning the trip, so . . . waiting that interval didn't significantly, even if it were cancer, disrupt her chance of being cured.

Q. How long does it take to perform a biopsy, could it be scheduled the same day and done or do you have to plan in advance for that?

A. . . . since I have an operating room right in my office, it's done the same day. But Dr. Jackson, I don't know if he has that ability to do that the same day.

Q. Now, in this case . . . you are . . . in stage two and the clinical examiner knows that.

A. Yes.

Q. And with that knowledge, would the biopsy interfere with the trip or is this something minor that she can have . . . and go on the trip anyway?

A. Well, if you do a needle aspiration biopsy that probably won't interfere with the trip. But in 1982 I don't think there was anybody in Madison doing needle biopsies. . . . Now, in 1986 or '85 just the thin needle biopsy we can do very safely in the office.

When Leo Hansen finished his last question, Bill asked Dr. Mackman if he would agree that Donegan and Haagensen were the two critical authorities on breast cancer. The witness agreed. He also said that when Bob did a needle aspiration, it didn't necessarily mean there was cancer. But, Mackman had to admit that in his deposition he had said that he doesn't do aspirations if there isn't something discrete. He said, too, that he assumed there wasn't a discrete lesion because Bob hadn't recorded its measurements, its shape—any of those things any experienced doctor would do.

Bill thought this testimony emphasized Jackson's own dereliction regarding patient record keeping. The implication of what Mackman said was that there *was* a discrete mass because Bob had taken a needle aspiration in March 1982. However, there were no records of such a mass. And in November 1983, when everyone recognized there was a discrete mass, there were still no descriptions—no size, no shape, no anything—in Bob's records.

We believe Leo Hansen's questioning hit a nerve on the other side. After Bill finished his cross examination, Steve asked:

Q. . . . is it Dr. Jackson or an experienced examiner against somebody directly out of medical school that's significant to you?. . .

A. Yes . . . it's the experienced examiner. . . .

Q. It isn't particularly because it's Dr. Jackson?

A. No, not at all.

When we recessed for the day, Bill said he felt that Dr. Mackman had become a character witness rather than a witness giving opinions based on medical science. We both felt pretty good about the way things were going.

November 22, 1985

I was feeling optimistic as we started the fourth day of the hearing. I was sure I could get through Bill's cross examination of Bob Jackson without much trouble.

The first few questions concerned Bob's credentials. He essentially repeated the information given on direct examination. Then Bill asked if there were "certain authoritative texts you rely on as part of rendering your care as a gynecologist?"

Bob said there were, that the texts were by Williams, Novak, and Danforth. Others were named, but Bill, I knew, had especially wanted confirmation that the book edited by Dr. David Danforth was one of those he relied on in his practice. That book contains a key article by William Donegan. Bill would bring it up again during cross examination.

Bill then questioned Bob about his treatment of me. Bob said there was a possibility of cancer being present in my breast. That was one of the reasons he ordered mammograms in March and June of 1982—to exclude malignancy as a possibility.

Incredibly, Bob said he did not recall my having told him in March that I had an "abnormality" in my breast. He said he felt something "different" in my breast in March.

Q. . . . I jotted down a note to the effect that if you had encountered a dominant mass, and I attribute those words, I am sure I would have written it down?

A. Yes. . . .

Q. . . . you indicated you would have written down its size?

A. Yes, I would have been more specific.

Q. And you would have written down the way it felt?

A. Yes.

Q. And you would have identified as closely as possible the area where you found that?

A. Correct.

Q. And because you didn't, you don't believe you found the dominant mass in March of '82?

A. Correct.

Bill then referred to the report of my March mammogram from Dr. Davis of Madison Radiologists, which showed there was a mass.

Q. Does Dr. Davis say clinically if a mass is felt you should biopsy—

A. He said if there were a mass, and I took it to be a dominant mass. . . .

Q. But his actual words that you used simply said mass, didn't they?

A. Yes, that's correct.

Bob said that the mammogram was neither positive nor negative for cancer but that "cancer could not be a hundred percent excluded."

Q. Is asymmetry one of the symptoms that frequently occurs with cancer?

A. True also with benign disease.

Q. Is there reference to asymmetry?

A. Yes. She had a benign disease.

Q. Doctor, what's the reliability of a mammogram, or what was your opinion regarding reliability of [a] mammogram at that time in diagnosing a positive breast cancer?

A. Quite good.

Q. Ninety percent?

A. Somewhere between 85 and 90 percent, yes.

Q. The converse of that would mean it would miss 10 to 15 percent of malignancies?

A. Depending upon whose reports you read, yes.

In answer to a series of questions, Bob said, "I am sure she had fibrocystic disease in March and June." He added, "It could have been mammary hyperplasia." (That is defined as an overgrowth of usually benign tissue.) He also confirmed that with fibrocystic disease the prominence of the mass is greater before menstruation.

Then Bill asked:

Q. Doctor, does fibrocystic disease often precede cancer?

A. With a number of women that have fibrocystic disease it certainly can. There are numbers of people with fibrocystic disease and numbers of people with cancer. . . .

Q. But . . . the fact that you have fibrocystic disease drastically increases the possibility that you will later have cancer, does it not?

A. Three times, four times.

Bill's next series of questions dealt with my next visit to Bob's office on June 29, 1982. Bob admitted that whatever he had felt in my breast in March was still there—same place, same size, same characteristics. It was the same breast mass.

Q. So you would have to assume, would you not, that the mass has been persistent for a period of three months?

A. Correct.

Q. And isn't it true that when a mass is persistent, that raises significantly the possibility of cancer?

A. No, not this mass.

Q. Well, I am saying generally when a mass is persistent, it raises significantly the possibility of cancer, does it not?

A. Not necessarily.

And then Bill confronted Jackson with the text by Dr. Danforth, one of the books Bob had told the panel he relied on in his practice. Bill offered a chapter by William Donegan, a contributor to the book. He asked the witness to read the following paragraph:

A. Masses and cysts are often transient, and cysts can usually be identified with needle aspiration. Persistent masses raise the possibility of cancer.

Q. When you were done in June of 1982, to what degree do you believe you had excluded cancer?

A. I thought I had excluded cancer in a very, very high degree.

Q. Well, 95 percent perhaps?

A. With the stability of the lesion and the improved mammogram, I felt I had ruled it out to a . . . very reasonable degree.

Q. Would that be 95 percent?

A. I would like to say so.

Q. In fact, you said so at the time of your deposition?

A. Correct. I would assume if you say so.

Q. And does that mean there was a five percent chance Ms. Chechik had cancer in June of 1982?

A. Yes. That percentage would leave a five percent chance that I was wrong.

Q. And similarly back in March we said . . . approximately 10 percent chance after the mammogram and the physical?

A. Ten to 15, yes.

Q. And so if we were to play that out in numbers, that would mean one out of 10 women with Ms. Chechik's symptoms who had cancer would fail to be diagnosed based upon the procedures that you used?

A. If you use those numbers, correct.

Q. And as of June of 1982, one out of 20 women with those symptoms would fail to be diagnosed to have cancer, is that correct?

A. Using those figures, yes.

Q. Is that a reasonably accepted medical figure insofar as excluding cancer as a possibility, Doctor?

A. It's basically that we would like to not miss any cancers.

During questioning about when Bob expected me to return for another examination, he said, "We monitor fibrocystic disease every six months."

Q. Now, she had a little greater abnormality and something that required more monitoring than just a general patient, didn't she?

A. No. She had fibrocystic disease. . . .

Q. You didn't think there was anything necessary for her to follow up as of June of '82?

A. Other than the usual follow-up for fibrocystic disease.

The next line of questioning covered my November 21, 1983, appointment. Bob confirmed that he found two masses, that one was in the axilla (the armpit), that it was approximately three by three centimeters as measured with his hand, that the lesion in my breast measured three to four centimeters, and that both masses were firm and discrete.

The defendant went on to say that that description was different from what he felt in March of 1982, which he had described as "rubbery." He also said that it was different because it was a dominant or discrete mass, as opposed to the diffuse mass he said he felt in March of 1982.

Then Bill asked a series of questions about Bob's procedures for record keeping.

Q. Doctor, did you note the size or the feel of this discrete mass that you encountered in November of 1983?

A. No, I did not.

Q. Is there any reference to its size?

A. No.

Q. And that would have been three by four centimeters?

A. Right.

Q. Is there any reference to the fact that it's firm and hard?

A. No.

Q. Is there any reference to where in the breast it's located?

A. Outer quadrant. . . .

Q. Any reference to where it's located within the outer quadrant?

A. No.

Q. A drawing of where it is?

A. No.

Q. Whether it's fixed or mobile?

A. No.

Bill asked if these weren't important facts to record. Bob answered yes and then said that he "would have had a memory about it."

Q. Doctor, your label of what you encountered in November of 1983 is that you encountered something ominous, isn't it?

A. Yes, the axillary mass. . . .

Q. Doctor, did you tell Diane Chechik that the findings were ominous that you had in November of 1983?

A. I am not sure. I probably did not.

Q. Did you tell her cancer was a possibility?

A. I did not.

Q. Did you tell her it was advisable to do a biopsy immediately?

A. On her return we would have to identify what these masses were.

Q. Did you tell her it was necessary to do a biopsy?

A. I am not sure if I used the word.

Then Bill returned to some questions about needle aspiration:

Q. Would you agree the standard of care is that when someone does not obtain fluid on a needle aspiration they must perform a biopsy?

A. I don't believe that.

Q. Doctor, do you want to turn back to your authority again, the Danforth? . . . Do you have that?

A. Yes, I do.

Q. Turn to page 1202. Would you read for me, please . . . the first full paragraph on the top of the right-hand side of that page? . . .

A. A biopsy is indicated if, number one, no fluid is obtained on aspiration. Two, the mass does not completely disappear after all the fluid is removed. Three, the fluid is obtained as bloody. Four, the mammogram is suspicious for cancer, or, five, the cyst reappears after an apparently successful aspiration. These signs would suggest a solid tumor which may be cancer or an intracystic or partially cystic cancer. . . .

Q. Doctor, does the Danforth text that you rely upon say a biopsy is indicated if no fluid is obtained on aspiration? . . .

A. Yes.

Q. Doctor, in your mind was what you encountered in November of 1983 in any way related to what the condition was that you saw in March of 1982?

A. I saw it as a new entity.

Then Bill introduced a surprise: an Aetna Life Insurance Attending Physician's Statement that Bob's office needed to fill out for my medical insurance. We thought it would play an important part in the hearing. Bill wanted to know if the signature, "C. Robert Jackson, M.D.," was Bob's. If so, we could enter the form as evidence in the hearing, but Bob denied it. He said his office receives these kinds of insurance forms, but that he personally does not respond to them. He said that the "insurance ladies" take care of them. He also claimed he did not know who had signed his name, nor if anyone was authorized to sign his name on insurance forms. We failed at this point to enter the form as evidence, but I knew Bill had one more witness who could make it possible to do so.

Bill went on to another issue. He asked Bob if Dr. Schultz and Dr. Price, who were to testify for the defense, were close friends of Bob's. Bob answered, "They are colleagues." Bill repeated the question, and Bob repeated his answer. Then Bill introduced a transcript from another proceeding in which Bob had referred to the two doctors as close personal friends. After an objection by Steve that testimony from another hearing should not be permitted, Bill won the right to ask one question based on the earlier testimony.

Q. Doctor, my question once again, have you on an earlier occasion identified Dr. Schultz and Dr. Price as close personal friends?

A. I have.

Several panel members questioned the witness. In answering Leo Hansen's queries, Bob said that in November 1983 the suspicion was "high" that the mass, with axillary involvement, was not necessarily fibrocystic disease. But he did no further tests because he wanted me to have a "good time on the trip."

Bill supplied information that I was in New York from December 6 to 13. Leo Hansen continued.

Q. You had 15 days . . . , so there was no urgency in scheduling . . . a biopsy before she left on the trip?

A. Not at all.

Q. What you are saying is you were attempting to accommo-date her?

A. Yes, without jeopardizing her.

Q. Well, if it was, as you say, a high index of suspicion, isn't it important for you to know that rather than waiting . . . three weeks?

A. It makes no difference in her outcome if it were positive or negative.

Q. Once cancer in the second stage is discovered, waiting three weeks is of no consequence?

A. No consequence. . . .

Q. As we sit here today, do you have any question in your mind but what she had . . . cancer in March of 1982 but it wasn't detected?

A. More than likely. . . .

Q. Mrs. Chechik says that on the 13th day of November [sic] she came back to your office and you cried together, the two of you, and she says you said I missed it. I don't know how I missed it, but I missed it. I am paraphrasing . . . but she said you had a conversation together regarding this in-cident, and when you were asked . . . by Mr. Caulum if this happened, my memory is you say I don't believe so.

A. I know I did not cry. I know that I came around and tried to comfort her. I know that I firmly believe that I have not been mistaken in my mind as to what has happened, and I did not say that I goofed. I did not say that I was mistaken. I did not say that at all.

Steve followed Hansen with:

Q. . . . You mentioned that . . . it's your belief that Mrs. Chechik had cancer in her right breast in March of 1982, correct?

A. Restrospectively I suspect the possibility of cancer is certainly there. . . .

Q. . . . do you believe, Doctor, was it clinically detectable?

A. I do not believe it was clinically detectable.

And that was the end of Bob Jackson's testimony.

Dr. Blake Waterhouse was the next defense witness. An internist at the Jackson Clinic and one of the most respected doctors in the area, he was the physician to whom I had gone for my insurance exam back in March 1983.

Bill had been worried about Dr. Waterhouse as he prepared for the hearing. He knew, of course, about the insurance physical. And he knew the defense was depending on Dr. Waterhouse to testify that he hadn't seen anything, meaning a lump in my breast.

Bill talked with Dr. Waterhouse several times in the months before the hearing. In May the doctor said, "There was something in the breast." He signed a statement to that effect. He also told Bill that my recollection of our conversation during the exam was correct. That was the occasion when he said he'd "defer to Jackson" in the treatment of the lump in my breast. In that same statement he said he *did not* attempt to diagnose it; "I deferred to Dr. Jackson's judgment and investigation." He said further that if I had returned he would have performed his own tests to render a proper diagnosis.

To Bill that implied that Dr. Waterhouse would have done something different from Jackson. He began to sound like one of our negligence witnesses.

Eleven days before the hearing opened, Bill went over to see Dr. Waterhouse. With him he took "Betsy"—a rubber breast with many lesions on it. It was a device used for demonstrations. He wanted the doctor to identify what he had felt in my breast, if possible. Dr. Waterhouse did find something in Betsy to fit Bob's term "diffuse." It wasn't an area. It was like a rope. Dr. Waterhouse called it a "fibroadenoma."

Bill was quite excited when he told me about this, because, he said, all of the authorities say if you confront what you believe is a fibroadenoma you must biopsy it because it is so close in its feel to cancer.

When he examined Betsy, Dr. Waterhouse had also said that what he felt wasn't a wide patch, but was well defined in some ways. His assessment that it felt like a rope was different from Bob's. He had told Bill, "you could feel its contours." It was one to two centimeters in width, about the size of a dime.

By the time the hearing began, Bill felt he could hand Betsy to Dr. Waterhouse if it became necessary in the course of his testimony.

Dr. Waterhouse began his testimony by confirming his estimate of the size of the lump. His testimony fit perfectly with Dr. Golomb's testimony of two days ago. Dr. Golomb said that if it was the size of a quarter when I had my surgery, it would have been about one centimeter when Bob Jackson saw it. And it would have been one to two centimeters when Dr. Waterhouse saw it. When Dr. Golomb testified he had no idea what Dr. Waterhouse would be saying this morning.

Bill then questioned Dr. Waterhouse about what he would have done if he had treated me. He said he would have requested a mammogram. If that had been inconclusive, he said he would have referred me to a surgeon or examined me again within six weeks.

Bill asked, "Why six weeks?"

Dr. Waterhouse replied that, theoretically, if it was fibrocystic disease, it would have been different on a six-week cycle.

Dr. Donald Price, an obstetrician/gynecologist with Associated Physicians in Madison, was the next defense witness. His testimony went as Bill had expected. He claimed that Bob had done nothing wrong.

There was one interesting bit, and it came out during Steve's direct examination. Steve asked Dr. Price, "How do you know if there's cancer?"

Dr. Price prefaced his answer with the opinion that the other doctors who had testified shouldn't have commented on whether or not Bob Jackson knows cancer. "If Jackson said it wasn't cancer, it wasn't cancer."

Then Dr. Price continued, "For example, the other day a patient came into my office. I gave her a routine physical examination. I examined her breasts, had her stand up straight, and had her palpate. I found nothing abnormal except when I looked at her. In looking at her breasts, there was a little dimple in one of the breasts. And I thought that maybe it ought to be looked at. So I sent her to the surgeon. Sure enough, there was cancer there that wouldn't have been caught. I'm such an experienced physician that I knew the little dimple said we had to do more."

I found Dr. Price's testimony enlightening. In examining his patient he found nothing abnormal. However, when he spotted a little dimple on one of her breasts, he immediately sent her to a surgeon. Bob could feel my lump, but I was told to go home.

. . .

After lunch Bill returned to the Aetna insurance form. Because Bob denied that the signature on the form was his, Bill needed another way to enter the form as evidence. Rose Althaus, office manager of the Aetna branch in Madison, was sworn in. She testified that the form with Bob's signature on it came from his office. Her statement was sufficient to enter the form as evidence.

Sidney Carpenter, my good friend from Salt Lake City, was scheduled to be our final witness. This slender, brown-haired lady, who is just about my height, looked great in her wine-colored suit. But I could tell she was nervous as she sat in the witness chair. I wasn't surprised. It's not a nice experience.

Bill's plan was to end on a high note with Sidney. Bill began by questioning her about our friendship and the circumstances of my visit to her home in July 1982. He took her through the scene on her patio the night I told her about the lump in my breast and about how I asked her to feel it. She stated what she thought the approximate size of the lump was and emphasized that she felt the lump for a "very brief period." She also said she was sure that what she felt in my breast was hard and had defined edges.

Questioned by the defense attorney, Sidney said she had been instructed in and is experienced in breast self-examination. In answer to a question from Leo Hansen, she described what she had felt in my breast as "abnormal."

The fact is that Sidney did very well under questioning by both attorneys, as well as by several panel members. She was almost finished when Leo Hansen asked:

Q. I don't think this witness narrowed it down to where it was in the right breast. Where did you feel this lump? . . .

A. On the outer side.

Q. Is that the right breast or the left breast?

A. You just said right.

Q. Well, I did, yes, but I am asking was it the right breast or the left breast?

A. It's the left.

Bill turned white. I wanted to scream. Of course it was my right breast and Hansen had just said so. Somehow we both managed to maintain our composure. I could not believe this—just when I thought we had a better than even chance of winning. I clutched my belt tighter than ever and prayed.

Bill, trying to minimize the damage Sidney might have done, asked:

Q. You took some time in answering that question. Do you recall specifically—why did you hesitate in answering whether it was the right breast or the left breast?

A. This isn't a very comfortable position. I didn't want to say something without thinking.

Bill put me back on the stand in an attempt to salvage the day. He wanted me to rebut Bob's testimony about his not wanting to upset my plans for a trip to New York in December 1983. Bob had testified that was the reason he didn't tell me he suspected cancer when I saw him on November 21. Luckily, I am a pack rat and I saved my airline ticket from what turned out to be a very significant trip. The ticket proved that I had not known I was going anywhere when I saw Bob that day. The date on the ticket was November 29, the day I decided to go to New York and the day the reservation was made.

I wasn't really ready for this second trip to the witness stand, and I talked too much. But Bill assured me when I was done that it was better than ending with Sidney. He realized how tough it was for me to testify again.

Sidney had left the room as soon as she was excused from the witness stand. When the day's session ended, I followed and met her in the ladies room. I think she knew something was wrong. I put my arm around her shoulder and told her, "Sidney, you were wonderful, but it was the right breast."

She was horrified, almost catatonic. She said she had been very nervous and flustered while she was testifying. I tried to assure her that it wasn't fatal; our case was too good to be wiped out by her statement. She confirmed my belief that her main concern was the fact that I had cancer, not which breast I lost.

Before he left for the day, Bill told me he was to blame for Sidney's error. He said he had not adequately prepared her for cross examination.

As I reflect on the day's events, I remember that since the mastectomy Sidney and I have never discussed which breast it was. Our talks have focused on the horror of this disease, our friendship, and the importance of survival. Besides, when she was facing me, it was *her* left side.

November 23, 1985

Only one witness was questioned this morning—Dr. Alwin E. Schultz. An obstetrician/gynecologist, Dr. Schultz is a kind, older man in a solo practice. He had been called as a defense witness, but he could not be present. His testimony was on video tape.

The crucial part of his testimony occurred when he was asked:

Q. So you are saying that your interpretation of this would be that they felt the same thing . . . Dr. Jackson was feeling back in March of 1982? . . . did the doctors in . . . December in New York feel the same thing as . . . Jackson felt in March of '82?

A. That's right.

Q. And it was in the same area, wasn't it?

A. Yes.

I was startled to hear Dr. Schultz's testimony. He was a defense witness, but his testimony directly contradicted Bob's. Bob had stated that what he felt in November 1983 was a new entity and not what he had felt in March 1982.

Dr. Schultz's testimony was a surprise, but Bill had an even bigger one for me. About halfway through the tape Bill casually turned to me and said, "Now I can tell you. You have a friend I call 'Deep Throat' who helped me with this case."

Shades of Woodward and Bernstein!

All he would tell me was that "Deep Throat" was a Madison physician who knew about me and my battle with cancer, that he was concerned and wanted to help. But he insisted upon anonymity. And he had directed Bill to Dr. Golomb. Bill would not tell me Deep Throat's name.

That left me speechless, something that doesn't happen too often.

Deep Throat, whoever you are: Thanks!

It was now time for the closing statements of both attorneys. Bill was first. He opened with the statement that during the hearing certain assumptions were made, assumptions agreed to by all the physicians in the case:

> One of those assumptions is that mammography should not dissuade biopsy . . . because mammograms can only pick up 80 to 90 percent of what are otherwise positive carcinomas. We know that there's a hundred breast carcinomas out there. Mammograms will only pick them up 80 to 90 times.

He reviewed testimony and literature that says:

. . . when you choose to do an invasive procedure like an aspiration, you've made a choice that if you don't get fluid, you're going to go ahead and biopsy.

He next pointed out that both sides in this case hired and paid experts to testify.

. . . And at times . . . the inference has been made that because of the association with the particular side of the case the testimony may be tainted. What is clear, however, is that the treatise testimony here cannot be that way. . . . nobody could go out and get someone to write a book or . . . an article for . . . this case. These treatises are . . . definitive statements of what medical practice is and what it should be.

He asked the panel to remember that the defendant had not rebutted even one of our treatises.

Several times Bill told the panel that it was our contention that Bob Jackson was negligent, that he did not "exercise that degree of skill that is available to him given the advanced state of medical science." He cited an array of procedures—in addition to biopsy—that could have been done. They included ultrasound, available at the University of Wisconsin where Dr. Jackson was a clinical professor, or simply checking me after my period.

Nicely put was Bill's statement that most of the testimony was "from Dr. Jackson's perspective." But, he reminded the panel, "don't forget there was a second perspective . . . that was Diane Chechik's perspective. Her testimony was a quarter size lesion that she could feel."

. . . Now, who's in a better position in this circumstance to know what it did or didn't feel like? The person whose body it is? The person who knows what her breast feels like? The person who knows what's there on regular self-examination? Or a doctor who does medical evaluations, routinely, an array of them as he said and now looks back on a chart and tries to tell us what was . . . there?

. . . I suggest . . . that Diane Chechik is very reliable when she gives the testimony of what that lesion felt like.

Bill returned once again to the Aetna insurance form. He summarized the previous testimony. Bob had denied that it was his signature on the form. Aetna office manager Rose Althaus had testified that Aetna had received the form from Bob's office. Referring to a poster-size blow-up of the form, Bill pointed to the words, "Diagnosis, right breast cancer." In answer to the question, "When did the symptoms first appear?" the form read "March 1982." Regardless of who signed the form, Bill argued, the information provided came directly from Bob's records, and that information persuaded whomever filled it out that Bob first saw me regarding cancer in March 1982. "That's significant," Bill said.

Bill next touched on the subject of needle aspiration, the procedure Bob used in my visit in March 1982.

He stated that the experts—Drs. Hecht, Golomb, Mackman, and Price—and the literature all say, one way or another, that you do not do a needle aspiration "if there isn't some discrete penetrable mass. . . . We know cancer was present. There's no question about it. . . . You heard Dr. Mackman say it. You heard Dr. Golomb say it. The literature supports it entirely."

Part of Bob's defense was that the mammogram showed nothing. However:

. . . the report that comes back from Dr. Davis does not say there is no cancer present. The mammogram report says there is an increase in density, accentuated on the right. There's bulging. Bulging being consistent with cancer.

Bill repeated Dr. Davis's suggestion that "if clinically a mass is felt, it should be biopsied."

Bill had been allowed 40 minutes for his closing statement. He still had a lot of material to cover, so he shifted into high gear.

. . . if Dr. Jackson had had a dominant mass, we know he would have put down the measurement. We don't know that. In fact, we know the opposite of that. . . . In November he has two breast masses. He admits they're dominant masses. He says he thinks they're cancer. Does it say where? No. Does it say the size? No. Does it say what it felt like? No. . . . It doesn't say any of those things. He doesn't write down the size if it's a dominant mass. He didn't do it in November. There's no reason to think he would do it in March.

I liked this next bit:

. . . You have to believe Diane Chechik before you believe Dr. Jackson. Which of the two of them would know better what was going on inside of Diane Chechik's right breast? Next, . . . forget about dominant mass. Forget about biopsy. Dr. Jackson had ultrasound available to him. Dr. Jackson had available to him the ability to call her back . . . 5 to 7 days after menses to see if the condition changed. Dr. Jackson had the ability to refer her to a competent surgeon to evaluate this. He chose none of those things. . . .

But, indeed, it's possible Dr. Jackson felt fibrocystic disease and Diane Chechik felt a discrete nodule. . . . She found a lump. That's why she went to see him. We know fibrocystic disease masks other symptoms. . . . If he gets the appropriate information, he can conduct the appropriate test which is to evaluate her when the fibrocystic disease would be at its minimum. I submit to you that that's a significant act of malpractice. . . .

What does Dr. Cody do when she gets to New York? That day he biopsies her right then and there. What does he do after that? Get on the plane, Diane, go home and have your surgery. . . . Cancer has that effect. . . .

Dr. Jackson didn't know that there was cancer in her breast in November of 1983. . . . And he says that she was going to New York, but we know that that's not true.

Was Diane negligent . . . did she return when she was requested? Three months to the day.

Secondly, she thought she had a second opinion. Dr. Davis as the radiologist. . . .

Third, she had every reason to trust her doctor . . . when you deal with the questions here, that indeed there was negligence. . . . What does that cause? . . . it clearly caused one significant thing. It caused a delay of treatment of 20 months. . . . That changes the diagnosis significantly. She goes from Stage I to Stage II.

Referring to one of the articles entered in evidence, Bill talked about a table showing life expectancies based on the stage of cancer when diagnosed. He pointed out that had I been diagnosed in March 1982 I would have had a life expectancy of 23 to 27 years. Instead I have only five years.

. . . It also caused her to endure chemotherapy and radiotherapy. . . . We also know that it caused a difference in her approach to this. Her angers, her fears have been intensified. . . .

Pain and suffering we talk about. Humiliation, physical and emotional pain and suffering, loss of enjoyment of the benefits and pleasures of life, that's what's gone on here. . . . The pain of the disease, the pain of the therapy, the pain of the treatment and the pain of knowing it didn't have to happen. . . .

Bill ended on that note. Very well put. He would have a short time for rebuttal after Steve's closing statement.

Steve basically said that Bob Jackson was so good he could not miss cancer in March or June of 1982. No doctor could be that bad. He tried to persuade the panel that Dr. Waterhouse hadn't found what I said was in my breast.

The defense attorney kept talking about "common sense." He told the panel they must use their "common sense" and not be bound simply by the evidence. He repeatedly asked if "common sense" tells you this doctor could make this kind of error.

His pitch essentially was: Do you think—with your common sense—that this distinguished physician, who has practiced for 30 years, who examines 10 breasts a day for diagnosis of cancer, would miss an obvious malignancy not once, but twice, in March and June of 1982? Steve said that Bob Jackson saw the cancer in November 1983. He asked panel members if they could believe that this doctor had failed to make the proper diagnosis in 1982.

. . .

After lunch Bill had six minutes for rebuttal. He began by talking about whether the burden of proof was on our side.

. . . what we're talking about there is the greater weight. This is not a criminal proceeding. This is not beyond a reasonable doubt. What greater weight means is that if you put the evidence of one side on a scale and you put the evidence of another side on the scale, and the evidence of one side tips that scale ever so slightly, it is the greater weight of the evidence. That's what we must prove here. . . .

Once again Bill raised the subject of expert witnesses.

. . . I assume that you'll understand that medical practitioners are not overly enthusiastic to testify against other medical practitioners. . . . Indeed treatises are in large part what one must look to. But nonetheless, Dr. Hecht from the University of Wisconsin did appear here and say he believed that there was malpractice. Dr. Golomb from the University of Chicago did likewise. These are individuals who . . . were prepared to come ahead and testify, and it wasn't based exclusively on an aspiration procedure. It was based upon the whole range of information that they reviewed . . . that drew them to the conclusion that there was negligence.

. . . Who were the experts on the other side? We're talking about associates, close friends, if you will, . . .of Dr. Jackson who came and testified for him. We're not talking about just the prejudice of being on one side or another. We're talking about a close personal relationship.

Then Bill took up the "common sense" issue. In reply to Steve's plea to use common sense in deciding whether or not an experienced physician would make these errors, Bill said:

. . . I submit to you that that experienced physician made exactly those . . . errors. If you look to November of 1983.

Yes, this experienced physician in the handling of Miss [sic] Chechik made errors. He let her out of his office in November of '83. . . . Dr. Cody biopsied immediately. Does he [Jackson] note the size? Does he note anything about what happens? And then look to December for just a minute. Is December the note of a doctor who has thought he's encountered breast cancer? . . .

Then Bill read from a poster-size card, a blow-up of Bob Jackson's record.

. . . Phone call from New York. Had breast problem there.

Then Bill said, "That's not true . . . Dr. Jackson. We know she had the breast problem before she went there." Then he read from the card again.

Checked out by doctor and sort of went bananas with it.

Bill continued:

She was told she had cancer. . . . This didn't say confirm my suspicion, I needed a biopsy. This said she went bananas. That's not the note of a doctor who examined somebody in November and concluded cancer. That's the note of a doctor who missed cancer in November of '83 and covered it . . . because he had missed it in March of '82 and June of '82. That's what December tells us.

Mr. Caulum also indicates that our case . . . is based on whether or not Diane Chechik was sent for a biopsy. That's not entirely true. It's whether or not proper care was rendered.

Bill went on to say that if, in fact, Bob Jackson encountered fibrocystic disease in my breast, he did not follow the accepted practice.

. . . An acceptable practice in premenopausal women is to repeat the examination after an interval of two to three weeks at a different phase in the menstrual cycle. Simple procedure. Simple. . . . Dr. Jackson did not employ that. And I submit to you he's negligent for not employing that. He didn't even write down when her menstrual period was to know the extent of the fibrocystic disease. Dr. Price has his nurse do that routinely. Golomb says everyone does that. He failed to do that in March. He failed to do that in June. He simply failed to do that. . . .

Dr. Jackson didn't use the simplest of all procedures . . . returning five to seven days after her menses. That's simple enough in March and June.

Bill's concluding statement brought the tears.

Now, to the last concept. Let's just talk about the reliability of mammogram. . . . Mr. Caulum said he could find literature that would say anything. Don't forget he didn't find literature that said something different than we submitted here. If he could have found it, he would have found it. But as to the literature we've talked about . . . it says 90 percent reliability. . . . Dr. Jackson said . . . 90 percent sure in March . . . that it was not malignant. 95 percent sure in June it was not malignant. And then recall the testimony of Dr. Price. Remember the little dimple story? He saw a breast with a little dimple in it and he thought it was necessary to go further to find out what it was. A little dimple. Little dimple. This isn't what Dr. Jackson confronted. He confronted breast masses.

He confronted something that is of significant concern. One in ten. That means if you go by . . . what Dr. Jackson did here, one out of every 10 women who walk in his office . . . with breast cancer . . . aren't diagnosed. Is that the advanced state of medical science right now? Is that where medical technology has us? It isn't one in 10. It's Diane Chechik. She's not a number. She's a woman. She deserved to be diagnosed. She's not just that 10 percent that I'm sorry we missed. She's a person. And he missed it.

Diane Chechik went to Dr. Jackson for treatment. She trusted him. She believed in him. She's coming to you for justice.

That was it. The hearing ended and the panel met—beginning at about three o'clock—to reach a decision. I was exhausted, completely wrung out. I hoped the panel would rule in my favor. I knew home was the best place for me to wait for the news.

The weather this week was gray and bleak. Today there was blowing snow, and it was slippery. The man I was dating drove me across town to the hearing this morning. Bill was going to drive me home. I was glad I had made that arrangement; I don't think I could have made it home on my own. Besides, I didn't want to be alone at that time.

We finally left the hearing room a little after three. As we were putting some papers and other material from the hearing into Bill's van, Steve walked over to where we were standing. He wished me well. He said he was just doing his job in the hearing and he hoped that he hadn't been too harsh with me. He said that it had been nice meeting me and that he hoped my health would be good. Then he took my hand and said, "Good luck, Diane." That was a classy thing to do.

We dropped some things off at Bill's office downtown and then he took me home and told me to wait. A lot of snow had fallen by this time—it was almost five o'clock—so I had to stay put. Bill said he'd call as soon as he heard anything.

Patience is not my long suit. But I'm waiting. I was supposed to go to a cocktail party tonight. Bill told me to stay home. If we won, he said, we'd have champagne at his house.

November 24, 1985

Every time the phone rang last night, I jumped. My date came over. We talked about the past five days while we waited.

At 6:30 the phone rang. It was Bill. His voice was very soft and calm.

"Well, did I win?" I asked.

He started to read from the panel's findings.

"Was respondent, C. Robert Jackson, M.D., negligent in rendering medical services to claimant, Diane Chechik? Answer: Yes.

"If you answer Question 1 'yes,' answer this question: Was such negligence a cause of injury to claimant, Diane Chechik? Answer: Yes.

"Was claimant, Diane Chechik, negligent for her own health and well-being? Answer: Yes.

"If you answer Question No. 3 'yes,' answer this question: Was such negligence of Diane Chechik a cause of injury to herself? Answer: Yes.

"If you answer Questions 2 and 4 both 'yes,' answer this question: Taking the negligence which combined to cause injury to Diane Chechik to be 100%, what percentage or part thereof do you attribute to: a) C. Robert Jackson, b) Diane Chechik . . . ."

"Bill," I said, "Did I win?"

"Just a minute. Do you have a pencil?" he replied.

"Come on, Bill."

"Wait," he said. In the same tone of voice he started giving me numbers to write down.

"Past and medical and hospital expenses? $15,000.

"Past loss of earnings? $10,000.

"Future loss of earning capacity? $70,000.

"Past and future pain, suffering, and disability? $300,000. . . ."

Suddenly they made sense. I screamed, "We won! I won!"

"We sure did. It was a five to zero decision," Bill told me. "The panel voted unanimously that Bob Jackson was negligent and that his negligence was a substantial factor in causing injury to you." He was talking excitedly. And I continued to scream, "We won!"

I won! With just a two percent chance of winning, I had beat the odds. What a wonderful feeling. I think I was walking at least five feet off the ground.

Now it was time to party. I told Bill we'd be over soon with the champagne.

I called Mom, the boys, Dr. Carbone, and Dr. Cody in New York. Dr. Pellett was at his farm in the country. I found that number and called him. I called Felice, George Bush, and Aunt Nish and Uncle George in Florida. I wanted to call the whole world.

While this was going on, Joel walked in with a bottle of champagne. Rose Althaus and Sidney soon arrived. We all hugged, kissed, and jumped up and down with joy.

I emptied my refrigerator and we carried everything over to Bill's. Other attorneys and several of the secretaries from his office were there too. We had a great celebration. It was a great victory. I felt better than I had in a long time.

Bill called Harvey Golomb and the other witnesses. We made sure that everyone involved in the case knew the result. There was only one questionable decision: the panel took $70,000 off my financial settlement because, they said, I should have gone to another doctor earlier. They call that contributory negligence. That annoyed some people, but I figured the other side had to get something. In the final analysis, Bob Jackson was found to be 80 percent negligent, and I was found to be 20 percent negligent. On this basis I was awarded $316,000.

November 23, 1985, was a day to remember. I won a sweet victory. But it isn't quite over. Each side has 60 days to appeal.

CHAPTER 7

December 21, 1985

The boys and I left Miami late today aboard a cruise ship. We're spending Christmas on the Caribbean. The cruise is a gift to Marc and Joel.

I bought a copy of *The Wisconsin State Journal* as we were going to catch our 6:30 A.M. plane to Miami. And there in the Metro section was an article about my award of $316,000 in the malpractice suit.

December 25, 1985

What an absolutely fantastic Christmas Day I've had. It's been a happy contrast to my past two Christmases.

First of all, I'm alive. I'm a very lucky woman. God has granted my wish—to live. It was worth the fight.

Second, I'm on this cruise to exotic islands with my two handsome sons. They are gallant escorts. The boys gave me a delicate gold bracelet for Christmas and with it a letter I shall cherish forever. Their handwritten note reads, in part:

December 25, 1985

Mom,

No, this isn't a Hallmark—they don't make them quite as informal as this. When you look over the horizon and all you can see is water, your mind gets cleared very fast. . . . It is refreshing and something you haven't had in a long while. This cruise is monumental in our lives. It celebrates a number of things. It celebrates us being together as a family of three. And even though we've celebrated Christmas that way for five years, this one carries much more importance. We've all had time to reflect upon the past and we've been anticipating what the future will bring. That's something we can't predict, but somehow we both feel that 1986 will be much more rewarding than 1985. It has to be. . . .

Mom, Joel and I love you very much and we appreciate this cruise more than you can imagine. It is beyond anything we could have had in Madison. Mostly, it's a wonderful opportunity to be together, even though we both know this family will *always* be together.

With much love and thanks
To an unsurpassed New Year
Your sons,
Marc & Joel

February 14, 1986

No appeal! At last I'm done with courts. After several rounds of negotiations between Bill and me and Bill and Steve, the other side agreed to the financial settlement announced last November 23.

This case is closed. But I still have no clear answer to my persistent question: Why wouldn't Bob Jackson diagnose my cancer?

February 19, 1986

This is too much. My lawyer Howie Goldberg called today. He shared with me some correspondence from Al's lawyer, Stephen Beilke. Al is taking me to court again, this time to get a restraining order to prevent me from using the settlement from the lawsuit for anything except medical and living expenses. Howie replied to Beilke January 23, 1986:

". . . I personally feel that any attempt on the part of Alan to restrain Diane's use of her malpractice funds would be contrary to law and a deprivation of her personal liberty. The funds that are received are because of *her cancer*, not for anything that Alan is entitled to. Surely, Diane has suffered enough without these kinds of added pressures. . . .

"Because of the obvious impact on Diane regarding your request and my response, I am not sending her a copy of your letter nor a copy of my response. I sincerely wish Alan would just leave Diane alone at this point in her life."

Beilke's response was dated yesterday. He said that Alan still wanted the restraining order, that "Alan recognizes that this is a very difficult period for Diane and he would prefer not to take any action, but he also believes that it is necessary to insure an equitable consideration during any discussion of maintenance." A court date was set.

Howie's response summed up my feelings exactly:

February 19, 1986
Stephen C. Beilke, Esq.
Kuemmel & Beilke, S.C.
301 N. Hamilton St.
Madison, WI 53701
    Re: Diane and Alan Chechik Divorce
        Case No. 80 FA 1335
Dear Mr. Beilke:
    You have got to be kidding.
           Very truly yours,
           Goldberg & Woods, S.C.
           Howard Goldberg

February 24, 1986

Bill, just back from a week of skiing in Colorado, called today with an ironic story. On the morning of February 15—the day after I learned there would be no appeal in my case—Bill was at the airport waiting for his flight to Denver. Someone walked by and said, "Attorney Smoler." It was Bob. Bill said, "Hi. How are you?"

Bill said, "Jackson glared and his kids glared. And I remembered your story about how you decided to sue him on the day he was headed to Vail and you were headed to chemotherapy."

February 27, 1986

Our court date has been cancelled. We signed a stipulation at ten o'clock this morning that Al will make no claims on royalties or profits from any book I might write, on any monies I receive from any closed corporation I control, and that he will no longer pay life insurance premiums for me. I gave up my maintenance payments.

That relationship is now truly ended.

Three hours later Bill called and asked, "Would you like to sign a couple of checks?" He'd received the checks for my financial settlement in the malpractice suit. There was lots of excitement when I endorsed those checks at two o'clock. Before the ink was dry on my signatures, I wrote one check to Bill for his fee and another for current expenses.

Before I left his office Bill told me that he thought my willingness to pursue the lawsuit was a "bigger risk than 99 percent of the people would take. I thought you were courageous as hell to take that risk."

Then I went to the bank and paid back the loan I had taken out to pay lawsuit expenses.

When I finally made a deposit in my savings account, the amount was little more than half of the original award. I didn't care. I was happy. For a change everything seemed right in my world.

The only check I haven't received is Bob's for $100. He lost his bet of December 12, 1983. I *did* have cancer.

March 12, 1986

Today is my birthday. And now that things have calmed down, I've had time to look carefully at my life since March 1982. I now feel driven to turn my journal into a book. I've begun to gather all the materials I'll need. I want others—especially other women—to reap some benefit from my experience. And maybe—just maybe—reviewing every-thing and putting it all together will help me find a reason for Bob's failure to diagnose my breast cancer.

March 31, 1986

The Common Bond Corporation (CBC) is now a reality. I registered this new corporation today as a non-profit group with both the state and federal government. I've long wanted to help cancer patients who come to the Univer-sity of Wisconsin Clinical Cancer Center. It's a lonely time.

My plans call for Common Bond to give a rose and a card to each patient beginning chemotherapy. Right now the cor-poration is inactive. I'll write my book. Then I'll be able to de-vote my time to CBC.

February 24, 1987

Today I returned to Snowbird, Utah, and my beloved mountains. After a few hours of skiing, I took off my skis and rode the tram to the top of one of the mountains. They gave me courage to fight for my life. Now I need courage to continue the fight, no matter what the obstacles.

In my mind's eye I imagined the mountains were covered with purple trees. What a magnificent sight. I felt close to heaven.

The slopes followed many directions, similar to my feelings since cancer. I took what seemed the *only* path, and fought for my life. The wrong path, the wrong decision, not being in tune with the environment—these can bring difficulty, danger, and even death.

EPILOGUE

July 28, 1987

Déjà vu.

Those words come closest to describing my state of mind as I write this last entry in my journal. Seventeen months have passed since the final settlement of my medical malpractice suit.

Why am I reliving these past three-and-one-half years? It started last Friday. A good friend called to tell me about an article in the morning paper. A malpractice suit has been filed against a Janesville, Wisconsin, doctor who failed to diagnose breast cancer in a 28-year-old mother of three. Her cancer had spread to other parts of her body by the time she was diagnosed by a doctor in another state.

That shook me up. I cried out, "Why is this kind of thing still happening?" I could not answer my question.

My phone started ringing again yesterday. Several friends called to tell me about a feature article on breast cancer that appeared in the Sunday paper. The subject was mastectomy versus lumpectomy in the treatment of breast cancer. The writer's use of "amputating the breast" to describe the surgical procedure of mastectomy was bad enough. But three paragraphs later he wrote that ". . . the fearsome disease that strikes one American woman in 10 could be curbed without mutilation."

I stopped reading right there. My eye would not go beyond that word—mutilation. It jumped out at me. I stared at it—mutilation. That's the word used most often to describe the act of cutting into women's breasts. Surgery on any other part of a body—female or male—is never described as mutilation. We talk about "removing" the diseased part. But with a woman's breast, it's mutilation.

It hit me! Mutilation is the same word used to describe the destruction of a work of art. Then I remembered words that Bob had spoken to me—"I could not cut into your beautiful breasts."

Was his statement to me an expression of his concern about mutilation? Were my breasts a work of art—beautiful objects to be viewed and savored? Would my beauty be destroyed if I had breast surgery? Would a beautiful work of art be mutilated?

Is this why Bob was unable to diagnose my breast cancer? Perhaps—but I'll never know for sure. I believe only Dr. C. R. Jackson knows the truth.

I've had a mastectomy. I'm not mutilated. I'm not a work of art. My breast is not an art object.

My mastectomy changed my body. It changed me. It changed my world. I still have cancer. But I'm alive!

APPENDIX A

Primary books and treatises entered as evidence in malpractice hearing:

1. Mann, Barry D., Donald L. Morton, et al. "Delayed Diagnosis of Breast Cancer as a Result of Normal Mammogram." *Archives of Surgery,* vol. 118, January 1983, pp. 23–24.
2. Danforth, David N. *Obstetrics and Gynecology.* 4th ed. New York: Harper and Row, 1982.
3. Haagensen, Cushman D., et al. *Breast Carcinoma.* Philadelphia: W. B. Saunders Co., 1981.
4. Donegan, William L. *Cancer of the Breast.* Philadelphia: W. B. Saunders Co., 1979.

Video tape introduced by Dr. Rudy Hecht in malpractice hearing:

Malignancy No. 1 in Women—Breast Cancer Management in the 1980s; a Continuing Medical Education telecourse; The Network for Continuing Medical Education, 1980; NCME 341.

APPENDIX B

The following forms, supplied by the University of Wisconsin Clinical Cancer Center, contain information about my chemotherapy protocol.

150

CHEMOTHERAPY

The information on the following cards is to help you better understand your chemotherapy. You may experience some, none, or all of the side effects. Your physicians and nurses are familiar with all of these side effects and will help you manage them should they occur. A physician is available 24 hours a day to discuss your questions or concerns.

Call (608) 263-8600, the Department of Human Oncology, for any of the following: (either the clinic secretary or page operator will locate your physician for you).

—Fever higher than 101°F.
—Shaking chill.
—Unusual bleeding or bruising.
—Shortness of breath.
—Severe constipation or diarrhea.
—Vomiting that continues 72 hours after treatment.
—Painful or burning urination.
—Blood in the urine or stool.
—Soreness of the injection site.
—Any questions that occur.

Your chemotherapy will proceed more smoothly if you:

Eat nourishing foods and drink plenty of fluids at mealtime and between meals.
Do not take aspirin (unless it has been prescribed by your physician). You may take Tylenol, Datril or Tempra if needed.
Tell your physician all the medications you are taking.
Check with your physician before having any dental work done.
Do not drink alcoholic beverages or do so in moderation.

NOTE:

1. Some drugs may alter your sexual drive or your ability to have children. If you are pregnant, be sure to inform your oncologist as some drugs may cause abnormal cellular changes in a developing fetus (particularly in the first three months of pregnancy). You may want to talk with your physician about birth control and family planning before beginning chemotherapy. You should also be aware that tiredness, fatigue or lethargy caused by chemotherapy can cause a decrease in sexual drive (this should only be temporary though).

(continued)

2. Left over chemotherapy medications should be disposed of properly. Liquids or pills should be returned to your outpatient oncology pharmacist or specially incinerated. Do not flush these medications down the toilet or sink. Unless otherwise specified, drugs may be stored at room temperature and always away from the reach of children.

8/81
This project supported by the Wisconsin Clinical Cancer Center and funded by NCI Grant CA 16405 and NCI Contract NO1-CN-55228.
Adapted from Yale Comprehensive Cancer Center.

CYCLO-PHOSPHAMIDE
(Cytoxan)

What It Looks Like:
White tablet with blue specks (25 and 50 mg).
Clear fluid after dissolved.

How It Is Given:
Taken by mouth or injected into the vein.

Common Side Effects:
Nausea and vomiting usually occur about 6 hours after drug is given
through the vein and may last 8 to 10 hours. When the tablet is taken,
nausea may occur throughout the entire day.

Partial hair loss may occur but is not permanent.

Nasal stuffiness, sinus congestion, sneezing, watery eyes, and running nose
during or immediately following injection of the drug.

Reduced blood counts occur 1 to 2 weeks after treatment.

Menstrual cycle may be irregular.

Less Common Side Effects:
Bladder irritation. This drug may produce burning on urination, or bloody
urine. **Adults** should drink at least 3 quarts of fluid (approximately 12
glasses of whatever you prefer including water, soda, tea, coffee, milk,
etc) during the day of the injection and 2 days after receiving the injection
of the drug. Empty your bladder frequently while taking the drug. When
taking the tablet, it should be taken early enough in the day to allow for
drinking large amounts of fluids and frequent emptying of the bladder. If
unable to drink fluids or pass your urine, call your physician. **Children** between 2-12 years of age should drink 2 quarts of fluid (approximately 8
glasses) and children under 2 years of age should be given 1 quart of fluid
(approximately 4 glasses) during the day of injection.

Storage:
Store at room temperature. Unused solution may be stored for 6 days if
refrigerated, but only in the glass vial. Do not store this medication in a
syringe.

8/81
This project supported by the Wisconsin Clinical Cancer Center and funded
by NCI Grant CA 16405 and NCI Contract NO1-CN-55228
Adapted from Yale Comprehensive Cancer Center

5-FLUOROURACIL
(5-FU, Adrucil, Fluorouracil)

What It Looks Like:
Clear fluid.

How It Is Given:
Injected into a vein or artery or topically applied. Occasionally, taken by mouth.

Common Side Effects:
Loss of appetite.

Diarrhea.

"Blahs".

Mouth sores.

Splitting of fingernails.

Dry flaky skin.

Metal taste in mouth.

Darkening of skin especially on face and palms of hands.

Watery eyes.

Nasal dryness.

Reduced blood counts may occur 10 to 14 days after treatment.

Less Common Side Effects:
Nausea and vomiting.

Thinning of hair may occur but is not permanent.

Skin rash.

Abdominal cramps.

Difficulty with coordination.

Special Precautions:
Do not stay in the sun for long periods of time because your skin is more sensitive to the sun, it may burn more easily than normal. Use a sunscreen lotion when in the sun.

Storage:
Store at room temperature. Do not refrigerate or allow to freeze. If drug is crystallized, have physician see package insert or return to the pharmacy to be exchanged. Dispose of excess solution properly.

8/81
This project supported by the Wisconsin Clinical Cancer Center and funded by NCI Grant CA 16405 and NCI Contract NO1-CN-55228.
Adapted from Yale Comprehensive Cancer Center.

METHOTREXATE

(Mexate)

What It Looks Like:
Yellow tablet (2.5 mg).
Yellow fluid after dissolved.

How It Is Given:
Taken by mouth or injected into vein, muscle or spinal fluid.

Common Side Effects:
Hair loss—thinning rather than complete loss.

Mouth sores.

Diarrhea.

"Blahs".

Reduced blood counts occur 1 to 2 weeks after treatment.

Urine may temporarily become brighter yellow after this medication is taken.

Less Common Side Effects:
Lung changes may occur. Report any cough, shortness of breath or fever to your physician. This will disappear when the drug is no longer taken.

Kidney problems may occur. Blood and urine counts of kidney function will be monitored on a regular basis.

Liver problems may occur. Blood counts of liver function will be done on a regular basis.

Nausea and vomiting.

Back pain while the drug is being given.

Special Precautions:
Report mouth sores to your physician immediately.

Do not take aspirin or anything containing aspirin (Percodan, Empirin) within 72 hours after receiving the drug without checking with your physician.

Do not stay in the sun for long periods of time because your skin is more sensitive to the sun; it may burn more easily than normal. Use a sunscreen lotion when in the sun.

If you have had radiation therapy, you may experience skin problems (i.e. increased redness or itching) in the irradiated areas. If this happens notify your physician.

Storage:
May be stored at room temperature. Excess solution may be kept for 30 days if refrigerated.

8/81
This project supported by the Wisconsin Clinical Cancer Center and funded
by NCI Grant CA 16405 and NCI Contract NO1-CN-55228
Adapted from Yale Comprehensive Cancer Center

PREDNISONE

What It Looks Like:
White tablet (5 mg, 10 mg, 50 mg).

Peach tablet (20 mg).

Colors may vary according to brand.

How It Is Given:
Taken by mouth.

Common Side Effects:
Stomach upset occurs in most patients. This can often be helped by taking the pill with an antacid, milk and/or meals.

Acne of the face, neck and upper chest may develop or worsen.

High blood sugar.

A feeling of well-being while taking the drug which may be followed by a "let-down" when the drug is stopped.

Difficulty in falling asleep.

Increased appetite and weight gain.

Less Common Side Effects:
Stomach ulcers may occur. Old ones may become active again or new ones may develop.

More likely to get infections.

Increased blood pressure.

Nervousness, depression (small percentage of patients have this side effect).

With long term use, a round face, increasing thickness of the back of the neck, abdominal obesity, cataracts, loss of muscle mass, more facial and body hair and weak bones may occur. (Most cancer patients take this drug intermittently. This helps prevent these problems.)

Special Precautions:
Patients taking prednisone for long periods of time should not stop taking the drug suddenly without talking to their physician.

Prednisone is available in many different strength tablets. Check your dose carefully.

Call your physician for a fever over 101° if an adult, or if a child for a fever over 102° while taking prednisone or within 6 months after taking prednisone.

8/81

This project supported by the Wisconsin Clinical Cancer Center and funded by NCI Grant CA 16405 and NCI Contract NO1-CN-55228.

Adapted from Yale Comprehensive Cancer Center.

156

TAMOXIFEN
(Novaldex)

What It Looks Like:
White tablet (10 mg).

How It Is Given:
Taken by mouth.

Common Side Effects:
Hot flashes.
Menstrual cycle may be irregular.
Bone or tumor pain (during the first several weeks of treatment).
Bleeding or discharge from the vagina.
Increased blood calcium during the first few weeks of treatment.
Report any increase thirst, drowsiness, constipation or increased
urination

Less Common Side Effects:
Nausea and vomiting.
Changes in vision may occur (with high doses).
Reduced blood count.
Hair loss may occur but is not permanent.
Dizziness.

Storage:
Tablets should be protected from heat and light.

8 81
This project supported by the Wisconsin Clinical Cancer Center and
funded by NCI Grant CA 16405 and NCI Contract NO1-CN-55228.
Adapted from Yale Comprehensive Cancer Center.

VINBLASTINE
(Velban)

What It Looks Like:
Clear fluid after dissolved.

How It Is Given:
Injected into vein.

Common Side Effects:
Reduced blood counts occur 1 week after treatment.
Partial hair loss may occur but is not permanent.

Less Common Side Effects:
Constipation.

Nausea and vomiting.

Headache.

Tingling, numbness or muscle weakness of hands or feet.

Depression.

Loss of appetite.

Fatigue.

Acne.

The drug can be irritating to the tissue if it leaks out of the vein. Tell person administering drug if you feel burning, stinging or pain while the drug is being given. If the area of injection becomes red and swollen after the injection, notify your oncologist immediately.

Storage:
Store in refrigerator. Unused solution may be kept for 30 days if refrigerated.

8/81
This project supported by the Wisconsin Clinical Cancer Center and funded by NCI Grant CA 16405 and NCI Contract NO1-CN-55228
Adapted from Yale Comprehensive Cancer Center

DOXORUBICIN
(Adriamycin)

What It Looks Like:
Red fluid after dissolved.

How It Is Given:
Injected into vein or artery.

Common Side Effects:
Nausea and vomiting may occur 1 to 3 hours after the drug is given and may last up to 24 hours.

Darkening of the nailbeds may occur.

Complete hair loss generally occurs 2 or more weeks after treatment begins but is not permanent.

Discolored urine (pink to red) may occur up to 48 hours after the drug is given.

Reduced blood counts occur 1 to 2 weeks after treatment.

Less Common Side Effects:
Heart muscle damage may occur. Studies are done before the drug is given and at certain times throughout treatment to assess heart function. Report any shortness of breath or ankle swelling.

Fatigue, weakness, the "blahs".

Mouth sores may occur.

The drug can be irritating to tissue if it leaks out of the vein. Tell the person giving the drug if you feel any burning, pain, or stinging while the drug is being given. If the area of injection becomes red and swollen after the injection, notify your physician immediately.

Special Precautions:
Do not stay in the sun for long periods of time because your skin is more sensitive to the sun, it may burn more easily than normal. Use a sunscreen lotion when in the sun.

If you have had radiation therapy, you may experience skin problems (i.e. increased redness and itching) in the irradiated areas. If this happens, notify your physician.

Storage:
May be stored at room temperature. Excess solution may be kept for 48 hours if refrigerated.

8/81
This project supported by the Wisconsin Clinical Cancer Center and funded by NCI Grant CA 16405 and NCI Contract NO1-CN-55228.
Adapted from Yale Comprehensive Cancer Center.

FLUOXYMESTERONE
(Halotestin, ORA-Testryl)

What It Looks Like:
Pink tablet (2 mg).
Yellow tablet (5 mg).
Green tablet (10 mg).

How It Is Given:
Taken by mouth.

Common Side Effects:
Masculine features may occur in females after using the drug for greater than 3 months, such as more hair on face, deeper voice, more noticeable muscles and veins, baldness and excessive body hair.

Increased sex drive.

Acne may develop or worsen.

Retention (holding) of body fluids.

Increased blood calcium during the first few weeks of treatment. Report any increased thirst, drowsiness, constipation and increased urination.

Less Common Side Effects:
Nausea and vomiting.
Occasional yellow or itchy skin which may indicate liver problems.

8/81
This project supported by the Wisconsin Clinical Cancer Center and funded
by NCI Grant CA 16405 and NCI Contract NO1-CN-55228.
Adapted from Yale Comprehensive Cancer Center.

THIO-TEPA
(Triethylenethiophosphoramide, TESPA, TSAP)

What It Looks Like:
Clear fluid.

How It Is Given:
Injected into muscle, vein, or artery.
Occasionally injected into abdominal cavity, bladder or space around lung.

Common Side Effects:
Decreased white blood count and platelet count which occurs about 14 days after treatment.
Pain at injection site during IM injection.

Less Common Side Effects:
Nausea and vomiting.
Absence of menstruation.
Tightness of throat.
Dizziness.
Headache.
Skin rash or hives.

Special Precautions:
Areas of previous radiation may develop additional sensitivity.

Storage:
Store in refrigerator at 35-45°F.
After solution is added, drug may be stored in refrigerator for five days.

This project supported by the Wisconsin Clinical Cancer Center and funded by NCI Grant CA 16405 and NCI Contract NO1-CN-55228.
Adapted from Yale Comprehensive Cancer Center.

PHOTOS

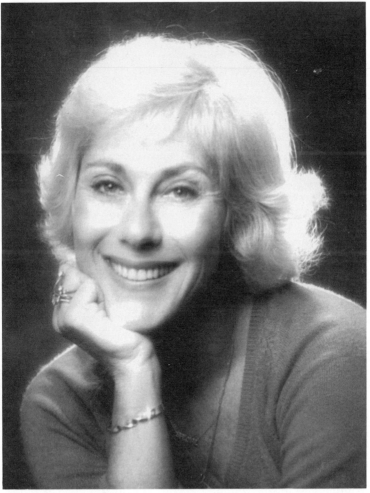

The way I looked in 1982. One of the photos used in the hearing.

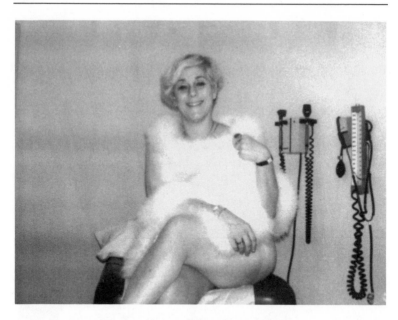

January 5, 1984—first day of chemotherapy at the University of Wisconsin Clinical Cancer Center—with boa.

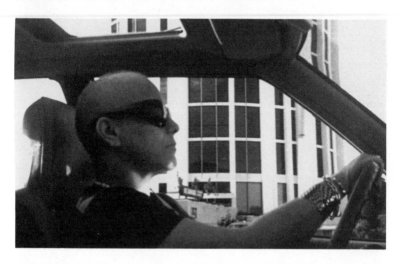

Driving in Madison, Summer 1984. Half-way through chemotherapy.

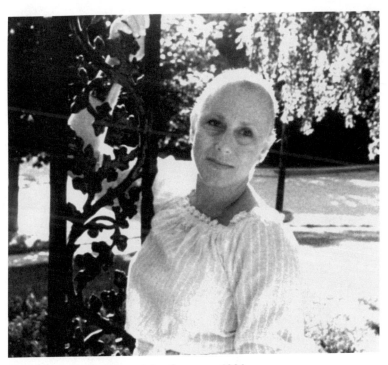

On my porch, before a date. Summer 1984.

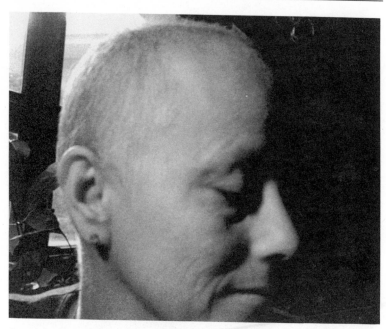

Second photo used in hearing. September 1984.

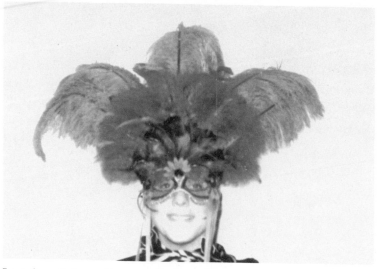

Last day of chemotherapy. Guess who?

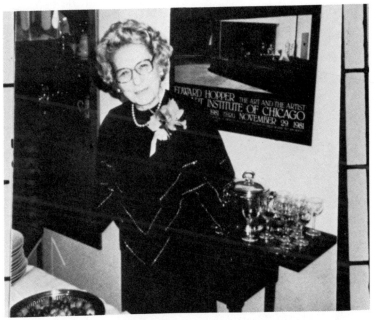

My mom, Dorothy Craig, on her 75th birthday, November 21, 1984.
Great lady!

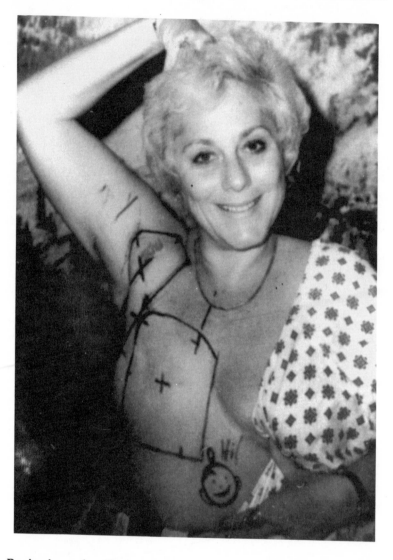

Beginning of radiation treatment after recurrence. Lines were guides for radiation therapists.

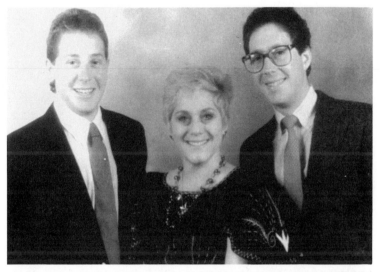

Christmas 1985 with my gallant sons. Joel on left, Marc on right.

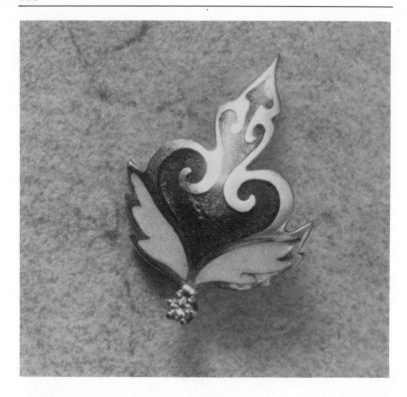

The Common Bond pin I designed with Kristin Anderson in 1984. The heart is for friendship and love. The wings are for hope for the future and the freedom to choose new horizons. The point reaches out to the sun for energy, the energy that helped me during my illness. I've given these pins as gifts to several friends. This is a photo of my pin, which is the only one made of gold and with a diamond at the bottom. The others are made of silver.